A Guide to Aging and Well-Being for Healthcare Professionals

This book provides practical evidence-based strategies that will help clinicians across a broad range of disciplines to address and discuss the main issues an aging person is likely to face and overcome if he or she is to maintain a sense of well-being as they age.

Based on an extensive body of research, the relevant up-to-date knowledge for each topic is concisely presented, followed by practical, concrete, evidence-based suggestions as to how a healthcare provider might acknowledge and create a partnership with their clients to help the person increase their sense of well-being. Each chapter contains a list of key terms, a summary, and case examples that illustrate in realistic and humanistic ways how a person might present the concern being addressed and intervene.

The specific challenges associated with aging that are addressed include: anxiety attached to an increasing awareness of mortality; retirement; the increasing number of losses of significant others; regrets; memory loss; the arrival of old-old age and feelings of loneliness, mattering insufficiently, and a loss of purpose; and finally, dealing with imminent death.

This book is suitable for all health professionals who provide clinical services or advice to older adults including physicians (i.e. particularly in the specialties of internal medicine, family medicine, geriatrics, and geriatric psychiatry), nurses, social workers, psychologists, physical therapists, occupational therapists, and audiologists.

Norman M. Brier (PhD) is a psychologist who was a Professor of Psychiatry and the Behavioral Sciences at Albert Einstein College of Medicine (AECOM). He has supervised hundreds of healthcare professionals in assessing and intervening with patients presenting with a variety of clinical concerns, and for more than 20 years has taught a class in patient-doctor communication. Dr. Brier is the author of a number of original articles and books. He continues to maintain a private practice in Bedford, New York and focuses especially on facilitating well-being in older individuals.

"Norman M. Brier has written a clear and concise guide for clinicians seeking to help older adults and their families to navigate the challenges of advanced age. The recommendations are realistic, pragmatic and empirically based. Both students and practitioners will benefit as they prepare themselves and those they serve to age with grace."

Gary J. Kennedy MD, Professor, Vice Chair for Education, and Director of the Division of Geriatric Psychiatry, Department of Psychiatry and Behavioural Science, Montefiore Medical Center, Albert Einstein College of Medicine

A Guide to Aging and Well-Being for Healthcare Professionals

Psychological Perspectives

Norman M. Brier

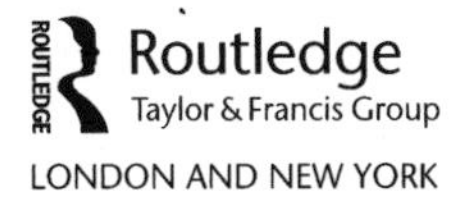

LONDON AND NEW YORK

First published 2020
by Routledge
2 Park Square, Milton Park, Abingdon, Oxon OX14 4RN

and by Routledge
52 Vanderbilt Avenue, New York, NY 10017

Routledge is an imprint of the Taylor & Francis Group, an informa business

British Library Cataloguing-in-Publication Data
A catalogue record for this book is available from the British Library

Library of Congress Cataloging-in-Publication Data
A catalog record has been requested for this book

ISBN: 978-0-367-43062-7 (hbk)
ISBN: 978-0-367-43049-8 (pbk)
ISBN: 978-1-003-00102-7 (ebk)

Typeset in Bembo
by Taylor & Francis Books

"The purpose of life is to live it, to taste experience to the utmost, to reach out eagerly and without fear for newer and richer experience."

Eleanor Roosevelt

In a rising wind
the manic dust of my friends,
those who fell along the way,
bitterly sting my face.
Yet I turn, I turn,
exulting somewhat,
with my will intact to go
wherever I need to go,
and every stone on the road
precious to me.

From the poem "The Layers" by Stanley Kunitz

Contents

Introduction

It is a common for people to want to have a "good life", a life that contains pleasure and meaning. As people age, however, what they consider to be a good life is likely to change, at least in emphasis. What matters and makes people feel good varies, in part, because people are more and more aware of the ever shrinking amount of time that they have to live, and in part, because of the constant reminders they receive internally and externally that their bodies and capabilities are declining. The awareness that they are "running out of time" is not only frightening. It can also have a positive effect. It can motivate people to view time as a precious resource, a resource that they have to "spend" carefully and selectively, and not waste; and with the realization of a relatively foreshortened future, a limited resource that they have to use more and more in the present with a focus on what is emotionally meaningful rather than on a potential, distant, hoped-for goal.

As will be described in detail, the likelihood as to whether a person will in fact attain a good life as they age is influenced by the degree to which they are motivated to: identify what matters most to them; evaluate and give significance and meaning to their experiences; and recognize, based on their past successes in coping with life's challenges, their capabilities, resources, and the degree of control they actually have (Folkman & Greer, 2000). It is also influenced by the degree to which a person can: maintain a positive attitude, and even when considering distressing events, see whatever potential benefits are also present; believe that they have sufficient personal control – that they can influence at least to some degree the outcomes that are important to them (MacLeod & Moore, 2000); and show "grit" (Duckworth & Gross, 2014) or a "fighting spirit" – a willingness to put out the effort needed to overcome the obstacles and setbacks that are inherent to aging, and reframe these obstacles and setbacks as challenges to be faced and surmounted rather than tragedies that need to be mourned, avoided, or feared.

Three key assumptions underlie the suggestions that will be offered to help clinicians assist people achieve and sustain a sense of well-being as they age. The first assumption is that while aging is characterized by decline and loss, gains are still possible. Thus, while people are likely to feel anxious and fearful at times, they can also experience happiness and contentment. The second assumption is that there is a great deal of heterogeneity among older individuals. While some older people will decline psychologically and physically relatively early, others will not. There is also a great deal of heterogeneity among the topics that older people consider to be important, meaningful, and pleasurable (Baltes & Carstensen, 1996). The final assumption is that successful aging requires flexibility and the need to rely on the processes of "selective optimization with compensation" (Baltes & Baltes, 1990); that is, people need to be selective in restricting what they do and strive for as they age, and make sure that their actions match their biological capacities, current skills, level of motivation, and environmental options. In addition, they need to be alert to the presence of occasions when they need to be flexible and adjust the strategies that they have used in the past, as well as their standards of success, if they are to maintain their sense of identity and self-esteem (Baltes & Carstensen, 1996).

In the first chapter, the components of well-being will be presented. I will focus specifically on how aging affects these components and a set of strategies that clinicians can use to help people maintain and enhance each component. In the second chapter I will first describe the major challenge to a person's well-being as they age – anxiety in the face of an increasing awareness of the limited time remaining to live and uncertainty about the nature and timing of the inevitable biological changes that will occur. I will then present ways that a clinician can help people cope with this challenge. In the third chapter, I will describe a second major challenge to people's well-being that many but not all people will experience, retirement, and in the fourth chapter present still another major challenge which almost no one escapes, the death of significant others. In Chapter 5, I will discuss the likelihood that as people get older and look back at their life they may experience regrets. I will then provide strategies that a clinician can use to help a person manage the negative reactions that may then arise so that the person can "seize the day" and use their regrets as a source of motivation to set and work towards achieving new goals. In Chapter 6, I will describe the challenge of age-associated memory loss and present ways that a clinician can help someone cope with memory failures. In Chapter 7, I will highlight the issues that are likely to be present as people transition from young-old to old-old age, and the effects of these issues on their sense of well-being. In Chapter 8, I will describe three additional threats to people's well-being that are especially likely to arise in late life – loneliness, a belief that the person matter less to others, and a loss of purpose, and in Chapter 9, I will describe the profound challenge to people's well-being that occurs when a person's health progressively declines and they may become aware of their imminent death. In the final chapter, I will present a review and synthesis of the ideas that have been presented. I will present case examples throughout the book to illustrate key ideas and strategies.

The concerns addressed in this book represent issues that most people as they age are likely to experience and need to manage in order to maintain a sense of well-being. Because most people as they get older are likely to have multiple chronic conditions, they will require the services of a variety of healthcare professionals including physicians, nurses, psychologists, social workers, gerontology counselors, and physical and occupational therapists. If a clinician chooses to use the knowledge contained in this book to help a person express their thoughts and feelings about aging, they will be offering an immensely valuable service.

As a famous psychologist stated, to face these issues is like "staring at the sun" (Yalom, 2008); to discuss a person's inevitable bodily decline, and especially their mortality, is difficult not only for the person expressing these concerns but for the clinician as well. As a result, many clinicians either avoid addressing these topics or, if they are addressed, they are discussed only superficially.

Thus, when a clinician acknowledges the person's concerns and does so with sensitivity and compassion, the clinician creates an opportunity for the person to feel both heard and understood – to view what are often private concerns as normal, and through the discussion, acquire both a language and a framework to better comprehend what they are feeling and thinking. As a consequence, the clinician will have increased the likelihood that the person will be more self-aware, clearer about what matters most to him or her, better able to prioritize and exert personal control, problem-solve, and experience pleasure and life satisfaction.

Chapter 1

Aging and well-being

Part one: A selective review of the literature in regard to the "nutrients" that people as they age need to "digest" in order to maintain and enhance their sense of well-being

Overview

When people are asked the question, "what makes me feel good?", their answers generally fall either into one, or both, of two broad categories. The first category, often labeled optimal psychological functioning, includes people who respond to the question by saying they have a sense of well-being when they feel that they are "actualized" and engaged. They feel good because they believe that they will continue to grow and develop, and as a result, feel they are "fully functioning" and all they can be. They perceive their life as satisfying, in large part, because they view the things they do as having purpose and meaning (Ryan & Deci, 2001; Maslow, 1971; Feeney & Collins, 2015). The second category, typically labeled happiness, includes people who respond to the question by saying that they have a sense of well-being when they feel what they consider to be a satisfactory amount of pleasurable sensations, emotions, and thoughts (e.g. when they eat food that they experience as tasty; when they are sexually stimulated; when they listen to music and perceive it as beautiful), and when they only infrequently feel such negative emotions and thoughts as anxiety and depression (Lyubomirsky, 2008; Seligman, Steen, Park, & Peterson, 2005).

When researchers measure well-being, they use these categories of optimal psychological functioning and happiness and study the factors that influence the degree to which people rate their life as satisfying and the degree to which people rate the amount of positive and negative emotions that they experience (Diener, Suh, Lucas, & Smith, 1999). Based on this research, people generally report a high degree of subjective well-being especially when they see their life as meaningful (based on their belief that they are achieving what they perceive to be important life or personal goals); engage in activities that they experience hedonically as pleasurable; are able to maintain a positive focus most of the time; have social interactions that they feel are gratifying; and see themselves as self-reliant and efficacious.

To consider the factors that contribute to well-being in more depth, the findings from these research studies will be used to delineate seven distinct elements of well-being. Organizing the data in this way, people as they age are more likely to report a sense of well-being if they: (1) can articulate and work towards a life purpose; (2) have a positive outlook; (3) experience pleasure; (4) have and are able to maintain close, supportive relationships; (5) have adequate self-esteem; (6) experience personal control; and (7) experience personal growth (Ryff, 1989; Seligman, 2011; Feeney & Collins, 2015).

By dividing up the two broad categories of well-being into these seven distinct elements we now have a framework that clinicians can use to help people as they age set goals and gauge their progress in achieving these goals. These categories therefore can be viewed as "targets" or aspirations that can help a person articulate what they need to strive for as they age in order to maintain or enhance their sense of well-being.

In the pages that follow, each of these elements will be further detailed.

Subjective well-being and purpose in life

As noted, people are more likely to have a sense of well-being and be satisfied with their life when they feel that what they have done and are doing is valuable and has significance (Baumeister, 1991). A person's need to identify what they feel is "satisfying" is likely to increase in importance as they age and are more conscious of how they will spend the precious supply of limited time that they now have remaining. Thus, with the perception that their time is becoming increasingly limited, a person is more likely to feel pressured to answer such questions as: Am I meaningfully using and apportioning the time that I have? Am I using the time that I have to do things that I consider valuable and important; and, is the way that others see how I am spending my time in keeping with how I want others to see and remember me?

Some people may be very self-aware and quickly able to identify what matters most to them - to easily identify the things that they attached special value and importance to (e.g. being with and feeling loved by their grandchildren; sharing their acquired knowledge and expertise with others; being able to recognize the times and activities that they feel are worthwhile) (Baumeister, 1991). The majority of people, however, are likely to have to carefully reflect on and review their past experiences, interests, and beliefs in order to adequately answer the question of what gives their life meaning.

As part of reflecting on and clarifying what matters most to them, a person might review the menu of life purposes that are typically identified by the majority of people in their cultural group. In western culture, for example, people generally view their life as purposeful when they are altruistic and self-transcendent (i.e. when they give to others and feel they are helping others, often by participating in "good" causes that are not primarily focused on their personal interests); morally good (i.e. they engage in actions they and others think are right and justifiable); creative (i.e. they produce something that they perceive has value); living life fully (i.e. they are curious and engaged), and self-actualized (i.e. they believe that they are achieving their potential and are able to experience a sense of personal growth); and lastly, efficacious (i.e. they experience feelings of competence and control) (Reker, Peacock, & Wong, 1987).

Once a person has identified their life purposes, they now have a set of goals that they can use to organize how they spend their time, a framework as they get older to decide how to allocate their resources (e.g. money); prioritize what they do; and monitor the degree to which they are achieving their goals so they can know when they need to put out more effort or revise their goals if what they have considered important and valuable changes (Baltes, 1997; Baltes & Baltes, 1990; McKnight & Kashdan, 2009).

Thus, by having greater clarity in knowing what they want to achieve, a person is more likely to be motivated to exert effort and expect success (Brier, 2015), and more likely to overcome adversity because they now have a rationale that provides them with an explanation as to why they should push forward during difficult times (Folkman & Greer, 2000). Finally, with greater clarity, a person is also more likely to be able to judge if they are acting in accordance with what they have deemed important, and know what they now have to change in order for their actions to be congruent with what most matters to them if they conclude they are not (McKnight & Kashdan, 2009).

Well-being, pleasure, and positivity

The second essential ingredient that is needed to maintain a sense of well-being is both the presence of a sufficient degree of pleasurable moments during which a person feels enjoyment, enthusiasm, stimulation, energy, and engagement on the one hand, and on the other, the absence of a high number of displeasing or negative moments during which a person feels angry, guilty, sad, or fearful (Seligman, 2002).

In addition to feelings, a person's attitudes or beliefs also contribute to their sense of well-being. People are more likely to experience a sense of well-being if they maintain a positive attitude in the face of the losses and physical decline that is inherent to aging (Diener, 1984). The key elements of a positive attitude include: the degree to which a person has optimistic expectations, is able to appreciate the value, meaningfulness, or importance of the major aspects of his or her life, and, especially, if the person is able to focus on what they see as sources of gratitude so that they are thankful and do not take for granted unanticipated "positives" when they arise (Huta & Ryan, 2010). A main obstacle to attaining and maintaining a positive attitude as people age are regrets, which tend to arise when people look backwards and focus on experiences that cause them to feel sad, remorseful, disappointed, guilty, or ashamed (Baltes & Smith, 1990).

Finally, people's ability to be calm also impacts the degree to which they can maintain a positive attitude. The ability to be calm is primarily influenced by expectations. People are more likely to maintain a state of calmness and a positive attitude when they do not expect to obtain what is no longer possible or under their personal control; view what they have and enjoy as good enough and satisfying; and resist comparing what they now have with what they have had in the past or with what others have (Diener & Ryan, 2009).

Well-being and close supportive relationships

Another especially important ingredient of well-being as people age is the presence of stable, emotionally close relationships characterized by affection and empathy (Lang & Carstensen, 1994). Intimate and supportive relationships allow people to feel cared for, understood, validated, and comforted. They reduce people's stress by providing practical assistance, advice, acceptance, understanding, reassurance, and encouragement. Further, in the face of the inevitable losses that people experience as they get older, close, supportive relationships help people feel safe, protected, and valued, which in turn, bolsters their self-esteem (Ryff, 1995; Seligman, 2011, Feeney & Collins, 2015).

Relationships with accepting and supportive "others" can also serve as catalysts, or sources of encouragement, that help people feel sufficiently confident to take risks and try new, unfamiliar activities that can result in personal growth. In addition, afterwards, they can provide a forum to share and possibly amplify the effects of engaging in these growth opportunities. Further, the feedback given in close supportive relationships can provide a means for people to perceive themselves as they might optimally be. As a result they gain encouragement to behave more in keeping with their ideal or aspired self (Feeney & Collins, 2015).

People as they age become increasingly particular about who they want to socialize with and especially about who they consider to be a close friend. More and more, they tend to prefer emotionally rewarding interactions, want to avoid emotionally meaningless ones, and do not want to have contact with casual acquaintances (Fredrickson & Carstensen, 1990; Lang & Carstensen, 1994). As a consequence of being more selective and with age, increasingly experiencing the loss of important relationships, the overall size of a person's social network is likely to shrink (Rook & Charles, 2017).

What tends to remain within this now smaller social circle are longstanding relationships, many of which may have at times existed for decades (Lang & Carstensen, 1994). These relationships are especially instrumental in contributing to a person's ability to maintain a sense of well-being. Through their shared history and memories, a person gains a sense of belonging and continuity; reassurance that they are still who they have always been; and recognition and validation of key aspects of their self-concept that they have used to define themselves across time.

Thus, these long-standing, close relationships can be viewed as a social convoy or a "posse", as in old television westerns. As pictured in these shows, travelers who faced constant threats had "protectors"; people who would circle their covered wagons when they were under threat, just as people's close friends surround and protect them whenever they experience hardships, such as when they are ill or incur a significant loss (Kahn & Antonucci, 1980). Thus, close friends can be considered a person's "safe haven" (Feeney & Collins, 2015) and their "secure base" (Bowlby, 1982). And within this smaller, secure, safe haven, the way people interact as they age also tends to change. With advancing age, people tend to act more benevolently towards people who they feel close to and be less concerned about maintaining strict reciprocity, seemingly to avoid conflict and reduce stress (Rook & Charles, 2017; Ryff, 1995).

Well-being, identity, and self-esteem

People's ability to maintain their identity as they age – to believe that they still possess valued personal characteristics that they felt have defined them and continue to be the same person that they were in the past – is another element of well-being that people need to experience in order to maintain a sense of well-being. The first and perhaps primary challenge to being able to see and feel that a person is the same as they were, as a person gets older, is the awareness of physical decline with age and increasing likely presence of functional, health-related impairments and medical illnesses. As a result, people are likely to feel that they are less physically pleasing than they were when they were younger and less physically competent (e.g. easily fatigued, less coordinated, and less agile) (Dietz, 1996). The second challenge is the likelihood that with life changes associated with aging (e.g. retirement) and a decrease in biological capacity, the person will participate less in identity-defining roles and activities or stop them altogether (i.e. parenting, employment, a hobby) (Lodi-Smith, Spain, Cologgi, & Roberts, 2017). A final challenge to maintaining a person's sense of identity relates to likely changes in social feedback. As people get older they may at times be viewed through the negative stereotype that is often attached to aging and feel that they are now seen as old and less able (Ryff, 1989; Fazio, 2010; Dogan, Toten, & Sapmaz, 2013).

Thus, as a consequence of these challenges, a person may become less clear about who they now are compared to who they were, wonder if in essential ways they are still the same person, and be at increased risk of feeling self-critical and self-conscious. At times, they may also become increasingly preoccupied with changes in particular personal characteristics that they have valued, considered to especially define who they were, distinguished them from others, and viewed as integral to their self-esteem. For example, if a person has always been proud of their mental quickness, they may become especially upset about the time that they now need to take to think through a problem, or if they had been and had received acclaim for being an outstanding athlete, they may become upset at their increasing physical limitations (Brandstädter & Greve, 1994; Sneed & Whitbourne, 2003).

People are more likely to successfully cope with these challenges to their identity and self-esteem and maintain a sense of well-being when they: are aware of the possibility that they may be extra-sensitive and try to carefully and objectively consider their reactions when upset or when they receive feedback about themselves from others (Robins & Trzesniewski, 2005); focus on and retain an awareness of the ways that they continue to have value and continue to elicit respect from others (e.g. how others continue to appreciate their knowledge and kindness); recognize and feel grateful for occasions in which they are able to feel capable and efficacious; and exert effort to be all they can be in the present (Paradise & Kernis, 2002; Ryff & Keyes, 1995; Seligman, 2011).

Well-being and personal control

The degree to which a person is able to feel a sense of personal control is still another key element of well-being. People as they age are more likely to experience an adequate sense of well-being when they feel safe, secure, able to predict what is to happen, and in particular, when they believe that they can influence issues that matter to them. As people get older, their sense of personal control is regularly challenged. In part, this is due to their increasing difficulty in influencing events in ways that they desire and in part due to the growing sense of vulnerability they have that comes from being more and more aware of the finite, ever shortening, but unknown life span that they have remaining (Schulz & Heckhausen, 1999). As one author has written, "Aging is foremost a process of living through changes that are largely beyond [a person's] control" (Baars, 2017a, p. 1).

When discussing personal control, it is important to distinguish the amount of control that a person objectively has from the amount of control that they perceive or believe that they have. As people age, the specific factors that contribute to a diminished sense of both a person's actual and perceived sense of control are very similar to the factors that have been noted in regard to maintaining one's sense of identity. They include: a decline in functional abilities (e.g. seeing, hearing, muscle strength); a decrease in the ability to maintain one's appearance as physical deterioration occurs (e.g. loss of hair, wrinkles, sagging skin); a loss of efficiency in biological systems (i.e. cardio-vascular, pulmonary, digestive); and an increase in the belief that others now perceive them as less attractive and vital (e.g. as old and less capable) (Schulz & Heckhausen, 1999).

Objective and perceived control affect well-being differently. The level of a person's well-being is more closely associated with their perceived personal control than with their actual or objective personal control. Thus, independent of the objective facts, if a person believes that they can influence an event, they are more likely to feel masterful and optimistic; and, if they believe that they cannot, they are more likely to feel helpless and pessimistic (Skinner, 1996).

Motivation plays an important role in the relationship between a person's sense of personal control and their sense of well-being as well. When a person believes that they have a great deal of personal control, they are more likely to expect to be successful, and as a result, more likely to exert effort, initiate action, and persist in the face of obstacles, setbacks, and failures. If they believe that they have little or no control, they are more likely to become passive, feel helpless, and when confronting obstacles, more likely to cease exerting effort (Brier, 2015).

Well-being and personal growth

A willingness to exert effort to experience personal growth is still another essential component of well-being. Because of a decline in biological systems and capabilities, regularly exerting effort to achieve personal growth becomes increasingly difficult as people age. Yet, personal growth is critically important in order to counter feelings of decline and the void that is likely to arise after the increasing occurrence of deaths of significant others who the person had participated in activities with. Thus, a person can feel that they are still able to "expand" or grow rather than "contract" or shrink if they enlarge their knowledge, abilities, and emotional repertoire and add new and satisfying experiences to their existing, familiar collection of life experiences (Ryan & Deci, 2001; Maslow, 1971; Feeney & Collins, 2015).

People who are able to experience personal growth as they get older are likely to demonstrate several specific characteristics. They are more likely to be open to novel experiences (Baltes, 1999). As a result, they create opportunities in which they can be curious, broad-minded, and imaginative; try out a variety of new ideas, values, and activities; are alert to things that might intrigue, interest, fascinate, and absorb them; and, most importantly, resist doing only what is familiar to them rather than keeping to their everyday routines and established traditions (Kasden, 2009).

Curiosity is a second characteristic that is particularly important if someone is to achieve and maintain personal growth as they age. Defined formally as the desire to inquire, investigate, or seek knowledge, curiosity is usually triggered by situations that are perceived as either novel, challenging, uncertain, complex, or puzzling. When curious, people are more likely to be energized to act differently than they have acted in the past. They "step" towards the unfamiliar; take an interest in aesthetics, such as art and natural beauty; select values and choices that matter most to them rather than choices that primarily matter to others; and seek experiences that intrigue, fascinate, and absorb them (Panksepp, 1998).

The degree to which a person is curious typically determines if the person will actually engage in a new experience when exposed to one. Feeling curiosity can be especially valuable as a person ages because it can reassure the person that in some ways he or she is still like they were as a child; they are still able to experience a sense of wonder and be fascinated when they discover something new (Berlyne, 1971; Kashdan, Rose, & Fincham, 2004).

The third especially important characteristic that is likely to affect a person's ability to experience personal growth is their ability to feel interest when involved in a potential learning experience. When someone is interested, they direct and selectively allocate a large portion of their attention towards the particular content of what has triggered their interest, and when they can maintain their interest, they are more likely to experience pleasure, which in turn increases their desire to focus more on what interests them (Hidi & Renninger, 2006).

At times a person's interest is especially strong and they experience a state of "flow" – they are fully absorbed, unaware of anything irrelevant to what they are focused on, and so immersed in what is occurring that they feel as if they are melded into, or part of what is the object of their interest. At these times they may also experience a peak feeling of enjoyment, feel that something significant, meaningful, and worthwhile has occurred, and feel a profound sense of personal growth (Seligman, 2011; Csikszentmihalyi, 1996).

While openness to experience, curiosity, and interest can facilitate a person's sense of personal growth and well-being, its antithesis, boredom, can reinforce the feeling that a person is stuck or shrinking. When bored, people are likely to feel dissatisfied, unhappy, disengaged, unchallenged, and uninvolved. They are also likely to have a heightened awareness of time and a feeling that time is passing excruciatingly slowly. At older ages boredom can be especially upsetting. Even though there is a pressure to make valuable use of the precious commodity of time, the person finds that time is "dragging on and on" and what they are doing is un-stimulating and lacking in significance or value (Csikszentmihalyi, 1975; Leong & Schneller, 1993).

While boredom is typically experienced as aversive, it at times serves an important adaptive function; it is a signal or "wake up call". It is an indication that a person has to exert additional effort to find activities that they can be open to, curious about, and interested in. When they do they are more likely to replace their feeling of being disengaged with experiences that are novel, stimulating, and meaningful (Bench & Lench, 2013).

The following vignette illustrates several of the key ideas noted in the selective review of the literature:

Maureen, aged 61, was divorced about ten years earlier. She has never had children and her main emotional connection has been to her mother, aged 91, who recently moved into a nursing home. In the ten years since her divorce, caring for her mother has been her main occupation, and now, without this as a central focus, she feels adrift and without a clear mission or role. Nothing at the moment seems to feel fulfilling or important and nothing seems to give her pleasure. After her divorce, she had to move from her home that had been located in an affluent area. As a consequence, she has lost touch with many of the friends that she had been close to and who she could rely on.

She now feels alone and very conscious of her age. On the few occasions when she does get together with acquaintances, she finds the conversation superficial, most often listens rather than speaks, and for the most part, feels as if she is invisible. She would like to date but feels that a man is now unlikely to find her attractive, given her sagging skin and wrinkles, and she is very conscious of the increasing number of ailments that she is experiencing. She believes that, like what happened to her mother, once you turn 60, it is "downhill". She thinks that there is little that she can do to influence how the future will go, and gloomily thinks that as she ages and her ailments continue to increase, she will be even less able to enjoy her life.

Part two: Ways of helping a person maintain and enhance the ingredients linked to well-being

The following ideas and strategies can be used by clinicians if a person raises any of the following concerns.

A desire to identify, articulate, and periodically update their life purpose(s)

If a person feels adrift and without a coherent sense of what they value and hope to achieve in the time remaining in their life-; if they are unable to set meaningful goals and efficiently apportion their resources (e.g. time and money) to achieve such goals, the clinician can explain that having an articulated sense of purpose is important. It makes it more likely that they will maintain their health and sense of well-being. In part this is the case because they will have a target they can use to assess the degree to which they are acting in alignment with what matters to them and can better direct their effort, time, and resources, and in part, because when they are aware of their goals, intentions, and the desired direction that they want to pursue, they are more likely to recognize and experience meaningful growth opportunities (Baumeister, 1991; McKnight & Kashdan, 2009; Windsor, Curtis, & Luszcz, 2015).

The clinician can describe several ways a person might be able to identify what most matters to them. The first way is after a crisis, such as the death of a child, the loss of a spouse, or the abrupt end of a long career, where what has just occurred makes salient what has prime importance in their life. A second more usual way follows from the fact that most people have only a vague sense of what is most important to them and are unclear about what direction they want their life to go. As a result, they struggle to identify and find words to articulate what it is that they might want to accomplish.

The clinician can reassure the person that they are unlikely to need to be creative; although the importance a person might attach to a particular life aim is likely to vary from person to person, most people's important life aims are not unique. People tend to select a life purpose that is very similar to what others in their cultural group select (Reker et al., 1987).

To help the person recognize a purpose that might fit what they feel is important to them, the clinician can review the life purposes, for example, people have identified in western society. They include: a desire to be altruistic and self-transcendent – to give to and be useful to others and participate in "good" causes that are not primarily intended to benefit their own personal interests; to be creative – to produce something of value that is relatively unique through their own efforts; to feel fully alive – be a curious, engaged participant in life; to be a good person – to engage in actions that are right and justifiable; and to be self-actualized and efficacious – fulfill their potential, experience personal growth, and competently and effectively influence situations that matter to them (Wong, 1989).

If the person feels that one or more of the life purposes that have been described are a good match, the clinician can offer to help the person be sure that what they have selected is actually a good fit by checking to see if what has been selected is consonant with what has mattered to the person in the past. Thus the clinician can suggest engaging in a "life review" or historical survey of past, major life choices (Butler, 1963; Butler, 2002). The person is asked to look backwards and identify critical "forks in the road", or major decisions that they have made over the course of their life, such as the decision to get married, take a particular job, or have a child. The clinician then can assist the person in identifying the motives, needs, and values that seem to have contributed to their making the choice that they did and assess how satisfied or dissatisfied they have been with that choice (Ryff, 1995). The clinician can then help the person juxtapose the values and needs that seemed to underlie these past choices with the life purposes the person has selected and together examine the degree of concordance between these past choices and the life purposes they have been selected.

The clinician can explain there is still another way a person might clarify their life purposes- by using "free association". The clinician offers to help the person remember significant, highly meaningful occasions during which the person either felt extremely happy or that their existence truly mattered. Using the occasions that came to the person's mind, the clinician and person can attempt to identify commonalities across these experiences; for example, to note if feelings of competence, appreciation, or being needed seem to be especially powerful elements of these experiences, and then consider if these same elements match what the person would still consider to be important needs or life goals.

If the person is able to identify a set of life purposes, the clinician might offer a caution. What matters to a person might change altogether or in degree at different points in time as they get older so that it is helpful to periodically reassess, especially after a transitional event such as retirement or the loss of a spouse.

Facilitating a positive attitude

Since, as people age, losses are likely to outweigh gains, a person may describe having difficulty either experiencing pleasure or having a positive attitude.

The clinician can explain that with effort there are several actions a person can take to increase the presence of positive emotions and reduce the presence of negative emotions (Seligman, 2002). Some of these empirically supported activities include the person writing a letter of gratitude to someone for something that they did that the person appreciated but had never previously shared, or especially, at the end of the day noting several good things that happened and the emotions that were felt at the time (Wood, Froh, & Geraghty, 2010).

The clinician can also mention that people are more likely to have a positive attitude if they have something positive to look forward to. Thus, the clinician can inquire about what the person might be looking forward to and if the person is at a loss, attempt to help them "brainstorm" using past events that they enjoyed or the experiences of others that they have known. If a desired future event can be identified, the clinician might add the caution that in order to maintain a positive attitude, a person has to adjust their expectations so that what they are hoping to experience at the time of the event is realistic and matches their capabilities to engage in the event (Holahan, Holahan, Velasquez, & North, 2008).

The clinician can also highlight another key element of maintaining a positive attitude as people age – the need to be selective, to carefully and thoughtfully choose activities and be ready to cease engaging in activities that are no longer as satisfying or pleasurable as they were in the past (Carstensen, 1995). Thus, to maximize positivity, people need to regularly assess the pleasure and satisfaction that they are obtaining from the activities they engage in so that they are more likely to have experiences they find valuable and pleasurable (Baltes & Baltes, 1990).

Another suggestion a clinician might make about maintaining a positive outlook is the importance of being self-aware and self-reflective – when experiencing pleasure and satisfaction, taking the time to identify what they are thinking and feeling and considering why these moments are valuable and meaningful to them. By recognizing and savoring such moments, the clinician can point out, people are more likely to see their life as fulfilling and more likely to feel that the life they are living is the life that they want to live (Watkins, Woodward, Stone, & Kolts, 2003).

Lastly, the clinician might mention that to feel positive, it is not only important to focus on what is pleasurable or satisfying but also important to minimize negative emotions. The clinician can explain that one source of negativity with age is regrets (Baltes & Smith, 1990; Torges, Stewart, Nolen-Hoeksema, 2008). As will be detailed in Chapter 5, a person is more likely to experience a state of well-being when they find themselves ruminating either about what they have done or not done if they try to forgive themselves – if they appreciate the context and reasons as to why they did or did not do something, and shift their attention when they catch themselves dwelling on what they now regret (Hill, 2011).

Helping a person maintain and strengthen close, supportive relationships

As people get older, they may no longer feel the degree of emotional connection they desire with trusted friends and care-giving figures and exert less effort to socialize (Fredrickson & Carstensen, 1990; Lang & Carstensen, 1994). The clinician might emphasize the critical importance of exerting effort to maintain the close relationships that are available and highlight that when a person does, they are more likely to feel listened to, comforted, reassured, respected, and supported, both emotionally and instrumentally (Feeney & Collins, 2015), and also more likely to experience lower levels of negative emotions (Antonucci, Ajrouch, & Birditt, 2013; Rook & Charles, 2017).

When encouraging social participation, the clinician can make clear that the level of a person's well-being is not primarily determined by the number of relationships that they have but rather by the quality of the relationships that they have. Thus, the clinician might help the person identify, prioritize, and strengthen the relationships that especially provide feelings of emotional closeness, reciprocity, and a sense of mattering (Carstensen, 1995). In addition, if the person complains about minor grievances that they experience in these relationships, the clinician can point out that since these relationships are so important to their feeling of well-being, they might consider ignoring or putting into proportion these minor annoyances and instead focus on the support and comfort that they usually receive (Luong, Charles, & Fingerman, 2011).

If the person not only is concerned about relationships but also hesitant to try out new experiences, the clinician can also point out that relationships with accepting and supportive "others" can be sources of encouragement. Talking over with close friends such ideas often might help a person feel more confident when considering taking risks and trying new, unfamiliar activities, and could provide a means to share, process, and amplify the effects of these potential growth opportunities (Feeney & Collins, 2015).

Lastly, the clinician might mention still another important benefit of exerting effort to maintain close relationships, especially longstanding ones. These relationships tend to bolster a person's sense of well-being by strengthening their identity or sense of sameness. The clinician can explain that when a person regularly shares memories with people they have been close to, they are more likely to have a stronger sense of continuity with their past. As a result, they are more likely to feel that they are still who they have been and less likely to be stressed because they feel, that at least in some important ways, they still exist in a familiar world (Brandstädter & Greve, 1994).

Helping a person maintain their sense of identity

When a person worries about maintaining their identity as they age – when they doubt that they still possess the same valued personal characteristics that have defined who they were and want to continue to be (Dietz, 1996), the clinician can explain that this feeling is relatively common and is usually due to physical decline, changes in appearance, changes in the roles that people occupy as they age (e.g. they are much less needed by their children compared to when their children were younger) (Lodi-Smith et al., 2017), and changes in the way that others now relate to them as they get older (Ryff, 1989; Dogan et al., 2013).

The clinician can add that the feeling of not being the same person as they age can also be the result of having less ability or satisfaction in engaging in activities that they have valued in the past, changes in everyday routines (e.g. being an early riser), and spending less time in familiar environments (e.g. in the outdoors) or with people who "talk and walk" like they do (Brandstädter & Greve, 1994; Sneed & Whitbourne, 2003).

The clinician can explain that one way they may feel they are able to be more "themselves" is to assess if they are spending a sufficient amount of time in activities that represent their interests and values. If they conclude they are not, the clinician can point out, they might consider modifying how they allocate their time so it is more aligned with who they are. As a result they will be more likely to experience a relatively higher level of pleasure and satisfaction (McKnight & Kashdan, 2009).

The clinician could ask the person, in order to help facilitate a sense of sameness, first, to describe those aspects of themselves that they feel have been relatively stable across time and situations, and second, to select from these characteristics, the ones they feel represent their essential qualities or "core" characteristics (e.g. being kind, athletic, thoughtful, caring, sacrificing, and assertive). Lastly, the clinician can ask the person in what ways with age these core characteristics may have changed (Baltes, 1997) and whether there are still ways the person can flexibly compensate to help maintain these defining qualities – to substitute alternate but related activities and interests for the activities and interests that they may now not be able to do or are able to be done only with difficulty, and as a result are experienced as much less enjoyable (Baltes & Carstensen, 1996).

The clinician might suggest, for example, that a person who has always viewed himself to be an avid reader but now is experiencing diminishing eyesight, in order to keep feeling like a reader, might listen to an audio version of a book; or, a person who has always defined herself as a musician and regularly played a musical instrument but now, because of arthritis, cannot play, to keep feeling like a musician, might teach others to play an instrument (Sneed & Whitbourne, 2003).

The clinician needs to point out that changes to aspects of identity, given the physical and intellectual decline that all people experience, are inevitable and that at some point no amount of substitution or compensation will be sufficient to maintain the ability to engage in one or more valued activities (Baltes & Baltes, 1990). The clinician can explain that the person at that point will have to face and mourn the loss of parts of themselves – to focus as much as possible on the core elements of themselves that continue to be present that they are proud of; aspects of themselves that they can still influence because they are relatively impervious to aging – qualities such as an expertise in a specific area of knowledge or a personal characteristic such as an insistence on being honest (Brandstädter & Greve, 1994). The latter, the way a person views making moral choices, the clinician can point out, is something that is both under their control, and something that can have an especially strong impact on their sense of identity and self-esteem – when a person acts in keeping with their values, with beliefs that they feel are right and important, especially when doing so is difficult, they are more likely to feel they are who they want to be and more likely to experience pride (Erikson, 1985).

Helping a person maintain self-esteem and personal control

As mentioned, people starting in the early sixties often experience a decline in self-esteem due, in part, to a deterioration in such physical functions as strength, coordination, and agility, and a decrease in their satisfaction with their appearance (Dietz, 1996; Robins & Trzesniewski, 2005). The clinician might try to normalize the person's concerns by noting that most people feel as they do, upset and disappointed, but eventually overcome their distress and recognize that "it is the way it is" (Neff, 2003). The clinician could also explain that a person is less likely to be distressed by these inevitable biological changes if they are willing to redirect their attention and selectively focus on what they can continue to do well and like about their appearance (Carstensen, 1995; Seligman, 2011).

People as they get older are not only likely to complain about their decreasing physical abilities and appearance but more generally about their lessening ability to influence external events to the degree that they wish (e.g. to lift an object, to travel long distances). The clinician can suggest that it is helpful at these times to reframe the issue of control and focus on a person's internal world, especially their choices, which they are still likely to be able to control. The clinician can point out that people are likely to have a relatively higher level of self-esteem and sense of personal control if they feel they are the decision-maker – the one who is able to select from among the options available what choice they prefer (Carver, Scheier, & Weintraub, 1989).

Further, by actively taking charge and asserting their point of view, the clinician explains, they are demonstrating to themselves and others that they are still in charge of their lives and still "masters of their ship" – that they are still autonomous and capable. If they have a physical ailment for which there is no immediate remedy, for example, as "captain" they can actively choose to search for another physician to help them manage the ailment; seek emotional support to manage their distress; or choose to accept what seems to be the reality, that there is no solution at present (Atchley, 1993).

The clinician may also mention the importance of developing an attitude of an acceptance given the fact that, as the philosopher Seneca said, uncertainty, change, and death cannot be avoided (Tornstam, 1989). The clinician can explain that, given the inevitability of situations arising that they cannot influence, including the losses of people that are important to them, a person's well-being is likely to be higher if they do not protest or fight against an occurrence that they cannot control, and instead, view what is occurring as inevitable or a given.

In addition, it is helpful for the clinician to point out that however sensible the idea of acceptance may be, for most people it is an aspiration, a wished-for attitude that a person can attempt but at least initially is likely to fail to fully achieve. Thus when most people are faced with distressing events that they cannot control, such as the death of a close friend, being diagnosed with a significant health problem, or no longer being able to perform a fulfilling activity that in the past has been important to maintain the structure of their lives and identity (e.g. driving), most people at first protest, rage, and feel angry about what seems to be the unfairness of life. Over time, the clinician can explain, people's emotions tend to settle down and they are often able to accommodate to "what is" (Cummins & Wooden, 2013).

Helping a person be intellectually, artistically, and physically active and engaged in life

As people get older, they may describe feeling that it is less and less likely that they will get to do certain things that they have wished to do, either because they no longer feel capable of doing so, or because they feel there is no longer sufficient time to accomplish what they wish. The clinician might explain that most people recommend that when older, rather than focus on far away possibilities, it is helpful to prioritize the "now"; so that if there is something on a person's "bucket list" they wish to do, they should not procrastinate. In addition, as part of focusing on the now, people should seek novel experiences that might provide opportunities for personal growth and resist keeping to activities that are familiar, routine, and traditional (Baltes, 1999; Kasden, 2009; Ryff, 1995). Further, the clinician can point out that by being open and receptive to novel ideas, values, and activities, people are more likely feel they are "expanding" rather than shrinking and more likely to feel that what they are doing in the time they have is valuable and satisfying (Brown & Ryan, 2003).

The following vignette illustrates several of the strategies that have been presented:

Maureen was asked to come to the nursing home to provide background information as part of the facility's need to develop a healthcare plan for her mother. After providing the needed information, the physician asked Maureen how she was doing now that she did not have to devote as much of her time to caring for her mother as she did in the past. Maureen chose to give a real answer and said that she was at a loss. She explained that she had not known what to do with herself for a long time and that caring for her mother justified her having no life of her own.

Outside of caring for her mother, she said, she did nothing of significance. While the physician empathized with her obvious sadness, he noted that she seemed extraordinarily passive, as if this was the way it is, and that nothing that she could do could make things better. The physician went on to describe his admiration for residents at the nursing home who were her mother's age yet still exerted effort to set goals, learn, and take pleasure in new activities. As he left, he said, "And for all of us the clock is ticking; so if you do not act now, when will you?"

Afterwards, Maureen felt both relieved that she had unburdened herself and appreciated that she was heard and understood but also upset at the criticism that she thought was contained in the physician's comments, even though she thought it was valid. She had basically given up on living. She was especially upset at the thought that she might not live as long as her mother and that she might be more like her father, who died at age 63. She wondered how much time she did have left to live and whether she was willing to actually have a life. She felt angry at herself and self-critical, questioning why she was passive and unable to do more for herself.

Feeling nostalgic, Maureen thought back to when she was about age 12 and filled with dreams. She thought she would be a writer and create a book series that children would love to read. Each day she would fill journals with snippets of stories. In college, however, instead of majoring in creative writing, she chose to be practical and took business classes, getting a job at a marketing firm, which she gave up after the tumult of her divorce and her move to a small apartment.

While still feeling motivated by the conversation with the doctor, Maureen looked online for a beginner's creative writing workshop, found one, and with tremendous apprehension, signed up. She had considered backing out several times before the start of the class but forced herself to attend. To her relief, several of the people at the workshop had life stories similar to her own. They had an unrealized early interest in writing that they wanted now to resuscitate. One woman in particular stood out. When going around the room telling about themselves, this woman said that she had also been divorced and that she too was looking for something that might feel fulfilling. Out of character, Maureen approached the woman, whose name was Alice, told her that they seemed to have a lot in common, and asked if Alice would like to get coffee.

Over the next few weeks Maureen began to enjoy the class more and more. It provided a focus and something to look forward to, and the writing assignments provided her with a task that seemed meaningful. In addition, she enjoyed what now had become the routine of going with Alice for coffee after class. As she and Alice got to know each other better, Maureen felt that they each provided something of value to the other – each listened and seemed to attach significance to what the other person was saying.

Now much more self-aware, Maureen realized how negative she had been and vowed to keep a diary as she did when she was a little girl. She would note what she appreciated and felt grateful for each day. She also decided to be kind to herself. Instead of beating herself up over what she had not done, she would be self-compassionate and remember how alone she had felt after the divorce, how shattered she was when going from being a married woman in a beautiful house and neighborhood to being a divorced woman, living in a small apartment in a middle-class neighborhood.

She felt proud of how she was now acting and grateful to the physician for challenging her.

Summary

Judgments as to what is meant by well-being as people age tend to fall into one or a combination of two main categories. People are thought to experience a state of well-being when they feel pleasure, see their life as meaningful, or feel their life is both pleasurable and meaningful. Seven sets of "ingredients" have been identified that seem to play an important role in determining the degree to which a person will experience a sense of well-being as they age. These ingredients include: having an articulated purpose for living; experiencing pleasure and positivity; possessing close, supportive relationships; maintaining a sense of identity; feeling adequate self-esteem; experiencing a satisfactory degree of personal control; and continuing to be active and engaged while in pursuit of attainable personal growth goals.

Clinicians can use these ingredients as goals that the people they are assisting can target and work to achieve. The primary strategies that have been described that clinicians can use to facilitate the attainment of these goals are assisting a person to identify, articulate, and continuously update their life purpose(s); carefully select and "optimize" the activities that they engage in, and while carrying out these activities, note what they appreciate and are grateful for; challenge regrets; maintain and strengthen close, supportive relationships, especially long-standing ones; work to maintain their identity and self-esteem, in part by acknowledging and accepting the inevitable decline they will experience in personal control; and engage in novel intellectual, aesthetic, and physical activities to counter feelings of stagnation and decline.

Chapter 2

Well-being and the anxiety about the awareness of limited time people have remaining

Part one: A selective review of the literature

There are two primary threats to well-being as people age. The first is an increasing awareness of the continuously decreasing amount of time that a person has left to live. The second is uncertainty; the awareness that a profound change is looming, yet no knowledge about when this change will occur or what form it will take (Greenberg, Solomon, & Pyszcznski, 1997). As a consequence, people are likely to experience a feeling of foreboding and can only look forward tentatively. Further, when they do look forward, they cannot be sure that they will be alive at the future time that they have pictured, or if they are, they cannot be certain that they will be healthy enough to do what they hope to do.

While people can never be completely free of the anxiety linked to these threats, their perception of "danger" and the anxiety associated with it, is likely to vacillate. People are especially likely to think about death and be anxious, for example, when they are ill, someone close to them dies, and when a significant life change linked to the passage of time occurs, such as retirement or a late-age, milestone birthday (Benton, Christopher, & Walter, 2007). These types of occasions tend to cause the person to focus on the fact that they are "running out of time", their physical capacities are declining, and the number of friends and family members who now have health problems or who have already passed away is constantly increasing.

Concerns about mortality tend not to center only, or even predominantly, on death itself. Rather people tend to also be anxious about the loss of dignity, control, and suffering that they anticipate; the likelihood that at some point they will need to rely more and more on others; and, as has been noted, the pain and suffering that is often associated with the end of life, at times, because of what they have witnessed of the dying process of others that they cared about (Hoelter, 1979).

Still another source of anxiety as people consider their mortality is the likelihood that a time will come when they can no longer do the things that they have enjoyed and which mattered to them (e.g., taking long walks) and a time when they can no longer fulfill a wish (e.g. travel to a distant location). Instead they may anticipate a future where they will be "trapped" and when life will contain many more negatives or losses than positives or gains (e.g. when they are frail, highly dependent, in discomfort, and constantly visiting doctors).

As a consequence of feeling uncertain, of being unable to predict and control the changes that the person knows are inevitably coming, they may become hyper-alert. For example, they may quickly notice and ruminate about new or unusual body sensations that they are experiencing and anxiously think that these changes signal the start of their physical decline or are an indication of a life-threatening illness. They may also become preoccupied with trying to guess how long they might live and, for example, regularly compare their age to the ages of genetically-linked family members who have died, the ages of people mentioned in obituaries, or the ages noted in life expectancy statistics (Pyzscynski et al., 1996).

The root cause: A fear of non-existence

There is an abundance of evidence to suggest that most people do experience fear when they directly focus on the fact that they will die (Greenberg et al., 1997) and that this fear may be amplified by whatever idiosyncratic concerns a person may have – concerns that are linked to their own personal histories and beliefs, such as being separated from loved ones or being in an enclosed space like a coffin. In addition to the fears triggered by uncertainty, a lack of control, and idiosyncratic concerns, the underlying fear that most people have is a fear of non-existence (Choron, 1974).

Thus, the core of people's anxiety about death seems to be people's inability to grasp or make sense out of the fact that they will cease to exist (Becker, 1973). Humans, unlike any other living species, are uniquely able to recognize and consider that at some point in time, and in some way, their life will end. They therefore are faced with the task of trying to imagine what will happen when inevitably this time arrives – when their physical self – their bodily functions – stop, and particularly, when they are no longer able to hear their "inner voice" and able to imagine a future (Burris & Bailey, 2009).

The nature and effects of uncertainty

Closely tied to a person's increasing awareness of death is their increasing uncertainty; although people are absolutely certain they will die, they are uncertain as to when this will occur (i.e. soon, in a year, or at the age a particular relative died) and uncertain how it will occur (i.e. suddenly or after a protracted period of pain). Thus, outside of occasions in which they are told that death is imminent, people cannot predict with any specificity the actual timing or nature of their death. At best they can develop a rough guess as to when and how they are likely to die, for example, using actuarial tables linked to their age, gender, and the nature of their health risks; or, if they have a specific, significant health condition that affects their longevity, they can develop a rough guess as to when they are likely to die based on the life span of others with the same condition.

Ultimately, however, no matter what a person learns from these attempts "to know" about the timing and nature of their death, they are likely to continue to feel anxious about what is never fully knowable. In addition, they have to grapple with the reality of the limits to their personal control – that there is nothing that they can do that would allow them to exist indefinitely and avoid death (Becker, 1973; van den Bos, 2009).

The need to develop a preview of what is to come

To cope, most people attempt to develop or adopt a set of beliefs that provide a "storyline" or preview of what will happen after they die and in this way lessen their anxiety about mortality. For example, people often identify a set of images, often comforting ones, that allow them to picture what they cannot actually know. In this way the unknown not only becomes known but at times even appealing; for example, a person might picture that after death he or she will enter heaven and be taken care of by a god-like figure, or be reunited with a deceased loved one that they have missed a great deal (Greenberg et al., 1997).

When people are surveyed and directly asked what they imagine will happen after they die, independent of the details of their response, most people express the belief that they will continue to exist in some way after their physical death (Burris & Bailey, 2009; Flynn & Kunkel, 1987). They seem to "fill in the blank" or the unknown to "see" what is ahead, and include within the blank the notion that they will be present after their physical death, directly, indirectly, or transcendently.

Thus, some respondents stated that they expected to continue to live on but possibly in a somewhat different form (e.g. as an angel), or without form as pure consciousness (e.g. as a soul). Others mentioned the idea of living on indirectly, for example, by being remembered and valued through what they have produced biologically (e.g. their children and grandchildren) or creatively (e.g. the photographs they have taken, the books they have written, the students who will use what they have taught them) (Lifton & Olson, 1974). Still others stated that they expected to live on transcendentally, without their inner voice or consciousness and in a way that is outside the limits of ordinary human experience. For example, they might exist as a cluster of molecules that would merge with, and be reabsorbed into, the molecules that compose the universe.

In effect, most people seem to do what Carl Jung, the famous psychologist, has suggested in the following quote to manage uncertainty and the unknown: "When I live in a house that I know will fall about my head in two weeks, all my vital functions will be impaired by this thought, but if, on the contrary, I feel myself to be safe, I can dwell there in a normal comfortable way" (cited in Lifton & Olson, 1974, p. 33).

Only a relatively small percentage of respondents did not provide a response in which they imagined "living" past their death. This relatively small group of respondents viewed death as an end point after which they, like all other living things, end and their existence ceases. Several people in this group also seemed to gain comfort by viewing death not as something new but rather as similar to the state of non-existence that exists before birth.

Inherent to people's focus on mortality is an increased sensitivity to the passage of time

As may seem obvious, when people focus on their mortality, on the limited amount of time that they feel is left in their lives, they are likely to be highly sensitive to events that signal the passage of time. They are more likely to notice the way the present quickly and irreversibly becomes the past, and how the amount of time that they have available increasingly becomes less and less. The result is that events such as the start of a new year, birthdays, or the change of seasons are often accompanied by a rise in anxiety, as well as at times a sense of anticipatory grief. For example, different than when observing the trees lose their leaves in the fall as a youngster and appreciating the vibrant colors, the older person may see the leaves on the ground and become anxious and sad, thinking that another season has passed and wondering how many more seasons they have left.

In addition, as a person ages, how to "tell time" also becomes increasingly challenging. Most people have learned to use clocks from a very early age to order events in a linear fashion, create a sense of predictability, and coordinate their activities with others. Yet, when people get older, what they are increasingly interested in is not simply knowing what time it is; rather, as mentioned earlier, they want to predict such things as the time when their body will decline and when they will die, information that is obviously not possible to gather using "clock time" (Becker, 1973; Baars, 2017b).

When older, using clock time to plan is problematic in still another way. Clock time has a steady, precisely-spaced rhythm in which each instant, as it passes, has the same value as the minute before. Clock time therefore cannot help people discern which moments in time are more important than others; therefore it cannot help people prioritize and allocate the time that they have.

Thus, instead of using a time-piece, to have a relatively higher level of well-being, people have to be self-reflective, decide what they think and feel is important and matters to them, and selectively apportion the time that they have (Cartensen, 2006). As noted when discussing the role of life purposes, to facilitate a sense of well-being people have to set and use their life goals to plan how they want to allocate their time and focus on pay-offs or gratification in the present rather than strive for long-term or delayed benefits (Carstensen, Isaacowitz, & Charles, 1999).

The following vignette illustrates several of the key ideas noted in the selective review of the literature:

Tom put down the phone. He felt very tired. He had just learned that his friend Frank had been diagnosed with a terminal illness; that would make the fourth friend this past year who had either died or would in the not too distant future. He wondered when his turn would come, and became even more anxious about the upcoming cardiology appointment. At last week's annual exam, the day after his 80th birthday, he was told that he had an atypical heart beat that needed to be checked out. Given what happened with his friend and the fact that he was now the same age that his mother had died, the person who had lived longest in his family, he thought that his "turn" was coming. Later, when discussing his worries with his wife, her attempts to reassure him by saying "everything will be okay", did little to calm him down. He was not sure what he did want her to say. Perhaps that she understood and that she too felt scared about illness and death. He both wanted the appointment with the cardiologist to come and dreaded that it was getting closer.

Just as he feared, the doctor told Tom that he had a cardiac problem; one that could be treated but not cured, and also told him that he was at increased risk of a stroke. In the days that followed, Tom was hyper-vigilant. He continuously checked the device that the doctor had given him to monitor his heart. Never having allowed himself to fully consider what it was about dying he was actually frightened of, Tom tried to find words to capture what most scared him. He realized it was the not knowing; he had no picture of what was to come after he died and did not buy the stuff that he had heard at church about heaven and hell.

As time went by, Tom's anxiety remained relatively high even though he was now taking a medicine that might delay a worsening of his condition. Thinking of what to do to fill his day now seemed more challenging. He felt that he needed to be productive – to not waste time, to do something, anything, rather than nothing, and to spend his time only with people who really mattered to him. He kept thinking about things that he could do to be healthier, but somehow, frightened as he was, he couldn't get himself to act very differently than he had acted in the past.

Part two: Strategies to maintain well-being as people experience a sense of uncertainty and are increasingly aware of their mortality

The following ideas and strategies can be used by clinicians if a person raises one or more of the following concerns during a clinical encounter.

Clarifying or helping people develop a set of beliefs or anticipations

As detailed in the previous section, a person's anxiety about death is lower when they can identify or develop a set of expectations about what will happen when they die, and especially, if they include within these ideas the belief that they will continue to exist in some form after their physical death. When a clinician is able to discuss and elucidate a person's beliefs in this regard, the person is able to make the unknown known and as a result is less likely to be fearful about non-existence; even though a person is likely to recognize and accept that their physical self will not exist, through this type of discussion, they can achieve greater clarity as to what they anticipate as well as reassurance that they will not simply disappear. Instead, as was described, they can gain comfort from the idea that they will continue on in some form (Kastenbaum, 2009).

The beliefs that a person identifies or develops, do not have to be rational as indicated in the Carl Jung quote presented earlier. People are likely to increase their sense of control and lower their anxiety if they can suspend logic and be open to ideas that some might consider illusions or magical thoughts (Case, Fitness, Cairns, & Stevenson, 2004). Thus, in keeping with Jung's idea, if a person is convinced that after they die they will enter a heaven with an all-knowing, protective and comforting god-like figure, their anxiety about death should be relatively low. The clinician can also explain that when a person is able to identify a comforting belief and share this belief with others and become part of a community of believers (e.g. by regularly attending a church service), they gain validation for their beliefs and their anxiety about death is likely to be especially lower (Rothbaum, Weisz, & Snyder, 1982).

Alternatively, the clinician can point out that instead of trying to "buy into" a comforting ideology about death, some people try to acknowledge their anxiety and accept their mortality. These people often attempt to deal with their anxiety about mortality, not by imaging a pleasing image, but rather by anticipating and visualizing how they would wish to act when the actual time of death approaches. If a person is interested in taking on this approach, the clinician might suggest that he or she read about others who faced death with dignity and, based on their readings, create an image of how they might wish to be when they imagine coping with dying.

The clinician can explain that they might imagine they are creating a movie script in which they star and the main protagonist is facing death in a way, for example, that both demonstrates self-respect and provides comfort to others who matter to him or her. The clinician might also point out that, after the person has developed a plan and an aspired set of images, they are likely to feel less anxious because they now have more certainty at least about how they want to manage what will occur (Brier, 2015).

Lessening anxiety and maintaining and enhancing self-esteem

When a person conveys that they are very anxious about death, the clinician can inquire if part of their anxiety is a fear that they will no longer matter to the people they are close to. If the person feels this may be true, the clinician can explain that this fear often lessens if the person can focus on ways that their life is currently meaningful and valuable. The clinician can point out that when people see their life has having significance and they feel "esteem", they are more likely to feel assured that they will be valued and remembered and, in this way, live on after their physical death.

The clinician can also describe how viewing their actions in a positive light, recognizing the things that they do that are good and valuable, may reduce their anxiety about death. When people are able to view what they have done and are doing as having worth and as conforming to their culture's standards of valued behavior, their sense of security is likely to increase and their anxiety is likely to decrease. This is believed to be the case because by "being good" they are likely to be reminded of the feelings of safety and protection that they might have experienced as children when their parents praised them for keeping to the norms and standards that their parents espoused (Greenberg et al., 1997).

In addition, the clinician can mention still another reason why, when a person's self-esteem is relatively high, their anxiety about approaching death is likely to be relatively lower – that is, they will be more confident that they can cope with threats, including threats to their health (Greenberg et al., 1997; Sherman, Nelson, & Steele, 2000). Thus, to help bolster the person's self-esteem, a clinician can carefully and systematically review with the person their past and present relationships and experiences and note and keep salient what the person has accomplished. In particular, the clinician can highlight that any enduring contributions that they have made are likely to continue on well past their physical death (e.g. paying for the college education of their grand-children; the teaching provided to their students). By focusing on these con-tributions the person can feel more assured that they have mattered and will continue to matter (Greenberg et al., 1997).

Helping a person accept what is inevitable

When the topic of death arises, the clinician might explain that many people use denial and avoidance to block thoughts about the possibility that they will die (Becker, 1973). The clinician can point out that the use of denial as a defense against death anxiety is not sustainable. As people age they are more and more likely to notice how their bodies become increasingly like the body of an old person and unfamiliar body "complaints" that frighten them and cause them to wonder if death is relatively imminent. In addition, they are likely to be increasingly aware of the deaths or serious illnesses of age-mates. The clinician can therefore make clear that people will continuously be con-fronted by indications of their mortality and, at best, can get only get tempor-ary relief when they attempt to deny what is an inevitable fact.

Thus, instead of relying on denial, the clinician can point out that acknowledging and imagining death is likely to be more effective and more likely to result in a relatively higher level of well-being and life satisfaction (Neimeyer, Wittkowski, & Moser, 2003). The clinician might use some of the ideas that were mentioned earlier to support this point or suggest ways a person might think about death so that it is less terrifying. For example, the clinician might suggest that instead of viewing death as a tragedy – an impending disaster with terrifying consequences – the person can try to view death as a gateway to a better life, or as a natural part of the cycle of life, in keeping with the idea described in the famous biblical quote, noted earlier, that "there is a time for everything; a time to be born and a time to die" (Klug & Sinha, 1987).

Other less terrifying ideas the clinician can suggest include the notion of viewing death as a return to what has already existed – the state prior to birth – and finally, at times, a preferred alternative to an often painful, debilitating existence that some people experience at the end of their life (Gesser, Wong, & Reker, 1987–1988).

It is often helpful in these discussions to use analogies and metaphors. For example, the clinician can present the often stated image of how people exist in a finite space and that death is a necessity to "make room" for new living things to be born. The clinician could also present a metaphor the person can use to imagine in a soothing way what is in store – to describe how some people gain comfort by imagining death as similar to stepping into a continuously flowing river, a river that has existed before the person existed, and a river that will continue to exist after the person no longer exists. The clinician could then highlight that when the person is in the river, they are one part of an endless procession of all the other people who have stepped into the river before him or her, and will be joined by all others who will step into the river after them. When presenting this metaphor, to further lessen anxiety, the clinician might suggest that the person imagine that, as the current is moving them along, he or she is relaxed and feeling weightless. Thus, instead of struggling or feeling tense, the person allows themselves to flow with the movement of the current.

Highlighting how a person's apprehension about death can be a prompt to live fully

The clinician can point out that anxiety about death can have a benefit; it can motivate a person to try to be self-actualized – instead of focusing on the shrinking amount of time that they have available, to seek challenges and fulfill their potential by utilizing their abilities as much as they can. The clinician can explain that when people use their apprehension about death in this way, their anxiety is found to be lower and their sense of well-being is found to be higher (Neimeyer, 2000; Wong & Tomer, 2011).

In addition, as mentioned, the older a person gets the more likely they will be selective in how they want to apportion their time. Thus, as part of an attempt to feel fulfilled, the clinician can note that it is important that the person thoughtfully choose tasks that seem important to them and which they are likely to enjoy and can offer to help the person think through which activities might fit these criteria. For example, together with the person, the clinician can discuss past experiences in which the person felt pleasure and satisfaction and see if any commonalities among these experiences can be identified. For example, the clinician and person could discover that the majority of these activities have included a great deal of interaction with others who are similar in interests to the person, involve an appreciation of art, or some form of novelty (Frankl, 1984; Yalom, 2008).

Assessing when anxiety about death and dying is excessive

There may be times when a person's anxiety about death and the uncertainty that they feel is so intense and overwhelming that it interferes with their ability to live (Yalom, 2008). If the clinician finds that a person is so worried about their mortality over an extended period of time and to a degree that they are unable to experience pleasure and satisfaction with things that have brought them pleasure in the past, a consultation with a mental health professional should be suggested.

The clinician would explain that the mental health professional is likely to use cognitive-behavioral techniques to help the person control their anxiety-provoking thoughts and, for example, might teach them how to switch their focus away from thoughts about mortality, reframe unrealistic or exaggerated fears, and show them how to focus on their breathing when a frightening thought enters their mind.

The following vignette illustrates several of the strategies that have been mentioned:

Tom's wife felt exasperated and guilty. She could clearly see that Tom was scared, understood why, and knew that he needed continuous reassurance that he was going to be okay; yet nothing she said actually seemed to help. She was worn out and at times just wanted him to man up and be quiet.

Sitting in the kitchen early the next day, looking through the local paper, she saw an advertisement for an upcoming talk at the local library entitled, "Staring at the sun: Acknowledging our mortality and facing our fears". She could not decide if this would be good or bad for Tom. On the one hand, hearing someone talk about this topic could make Tom even more terrified that he, like several of his friends, might soon die; on the other hand, maybe both he and she would hear some ideas that would help make things calmer. When Tom came down for breakfast, she mentioned the talk and to her surprise he readily agreed to go.

The speaker, a nurse-practitioner at a local nursing facility, acted as a facilitator. Instead of giving a lecture, she went around the room and helped people put into words how they imagined death, what they feared, and what, if anything, they did that either brought them comfort or made them less frightened. As they left the talk, Tom was quiet and, after a time, said he was glad that they went. When his wife asked him why, he said mostly because he now had words to help him figure out what had been bothering him. He went on to say that he had decided to speak to the pastor at the local church, something he had not done for many years.

When Tom met with the pastor, he asked him how he would describe what happens at the time of death and afterwards. The pastor then repeated the same unsatisfying ideas that Tom had heard when he regularly attended church as a youngster. Yet, the pastor did say some things that Tom thought had value. He talked of the importance, when trying to cope with the unknowns that lie ahead, of creating and being comforted by a positive hope of what may happen after death and to focus on what you can control in the present, for example, how Tom could better manage his anxiety.

Still anxious and feeling at a loss, Tom decided to call the nurse-practitioner, whose name was Sarah. He told her that he had enjoyed her talk at the library and asked if he could meet with her to discuss some of the issues that she mentioned. Sarah said she would be glad to meet and set a time for the next day in her office at the nursing facility. As Sarah listened attentively, Tom told her about his heart condition and his constant fear that at any moment his condition would worsen and he would die. He said that, even though others at her talk had come up with ways of thinking about death that were not terrifying, he, as of now, couldn't.

Sarah told Tom that from her experience of almost 30 years, many people who had his condition felt pretty much the way he did. She said that it seemed awful to have to live with this level of uncertainty and that all most people can do is try to not overreact when they feel a physical change. With their physician's help, she said, at best they can try to stay focused on the facts and most of the people she had come across seemed less frightened, if, as he was contemplating, they could picture what happens when you die in a way that was not only less scary but actually comforting.

Tom thought about his conversation with Sarah on the way back home and realized that in some ways what she had said was similar to what the pastor had said. He thought, however, that in contrast to the pastor, Sarah was a good listener and that it was a relief to let out his fears and especially a relief to feel that what he had said was not only heard, but heard accurately.

In keeping with what Sarah had suggested, Tom was able to come up with a comforting idea. He imagined that he would be reunited with his mother after he died and felt less anxious. She was the most loving, gentle person he had ever known. He pictured how, when he was a child, his mother would stroke his hair, soothe and reassure him, and as a result, as he had when he was a child, he felt safe.

Summary

A person's increasing awareness of their mortality and uncertainty about the inevitable changes that are in store are likely to challenge their sense of well-being. What a person does know with certainty is that they will die. What they do not know is how or when. What a person also does know that typically causes a great deal of anxiety is that "in route" they may suffer, lose their dignity, and be less able to influence events.

A clinician can help a person cope by helping them create a narrative of what is to occur at and after death – a narrative that supplies a "known" to fill-in for the unknowns that are looming, and particularly, for the unknowns attached to non-existence. The clinician can point out that most people select a variation of a narrative that exists in established belief systems, and some create their own narrative. In either case, the clinician can explain that in order for the narrative to be effective in easing a person's anxiety, it has to provide a "storyline" that counters their sense of uncertainty and reassures them that they will continue to exist in some form after their physical death.

The clinician can also mention that a small minority of people aspire to accept their mortality rather than create what they consider to be a make-believe story. These people attempt to view death as a natural part of the life cycle and view the limited time that they have remaining as a prompt which motivates them to make the most of the time that they do have available.

The clinician can also note that a likely consequence of being increasingly aware of one's mortality is a heightened sensitivity to the passage of time. More and more, people are likely to view time as an exceedingly valuable and scarce resource. As a result, they are likely to have a relatively higher sense of well-being if they feel they are using their time wisely and are seeking new experiences that are challenging and satisfying.

Throughout these discussions, the clinician needs to be alert to situations in which a person's anxiety about their mortality is so excessive that it regularly interferes with their ability to gain satisfaction or pleasure from whatever they attempt to do in the present. The clinician in this circumstance would discuss the importance of seeking a mental health consultation.

Chapter 3

A major challenge to well-being as people age

Retirement

Part one: A selective review of the literature on retirement and its effect on well-being

Overview

In addition to mortality anxiety, many people's well-being may be challenged by retirement, a major life transition that can be both stressful as well as potentially growth-promoting (Wang, Henkens, & van Solinge, 2011). Empirical studies are inconsistent however; some indicate that after retiring people experience a decrease in life satisfaction and an increase in psychological distress, others indicate that retirement has no deleterious effects, and still others report positive effects.

A large number of factors have been identified that are likely to influence the degree to which retirement will either positively or negatively affect well-being in the period following retirement. A person's well-being after retiring is likely to be relatively higher if, prior to retiring, the person had an adequate level of psychological well-being, financial security, and subjective health, and had experienced a great deal of work stress (Dingemans, 2012; Olds et al., 2018). In addition, a person's well-being is especially likely to be higher if the person's choice to retire was voluntary and planned, and the person had time to contemplate how they would manage events during the transition from working to not working (Dingemans & Henkens 2015).

Women relative to men have been found to experience lower levels of well-being following retirement; they are more likely to have more negative attitudes towards retirement than men, find it more disruptive, and experience a higher level of depression and loneliness after retiring (Kim & Moen, 2002). Finally, people's well-being following retirement is likely to be relatively higher if they have access to social and emotional support and can engage in satisfying activities once retired (Dingemans, 2012; Olds et al., 2018).

Recently, due to financial pressures, increases in life expectancy, improved health status, policy changes such as the elimination of mandatory retirement, and government work incentives that encourage people to remain employed, a larger number of people are retiring at older ages than they did in the past; gradually phasing into retirement by reducing the number of hours that they work at their career jobs rather than completely retiring; or taking a paid, often part-time, work position after they retire from a career job to supplement their retirement benefits (Davies & Cartwright, 2011; Tang, Choi, & Goode, 2013). In the United States, for example, the number of employees aged 65 and older who participated in the labor force increased from 12.1% in 1990 to 16.1% in 2010, and in the Netherlands the labor participation rate for the 65 to 75 age group doubled from 5.5% in 2003 to 11% in 2014 (Sewdas et al., 2017).

Whether retirement is primarily a source of tension or a source of benefit, voluntary and planned or involuntary and unplanned, occurs at a historically traditional time or at a later time, or is sudden or gradual, most people will experience their retirement as a milestone, an indication that they have completed a significant portion of their adult life span (Kim & Moen, 2002). As a result, and as highlighted in the last chapter, they are likely to be increasingly conscious of the passage of time, and increasingly focused on how they wish to "spend" the now increased amount of discretionary time that they are likely to have available (Osborne, 2012).

Retirement defined

Retirement has been formally defined as a person's withdrawal from a position, occupation, or set of activities that have made up their paid working life (Ekerdt & DeViney, 1990). Thus, by definition, retirement signifies an ending, and since people tend to retire when they are relatively older, thoughts about retirement are likely to be comingled with thoughts about mortality. Especially in the period following retirement, people are likely to experience such strong emotions as anxiety about what is to come, and sadness about activities and relationships that they will no longer experience.

In order to maintain a sense of well-being after people retire, they need to accomplish three specific tasks. They have to preserve and maintain their identity and self-worth; revise and reestablish routines and a life structure; and allocate the increased discretionary time that is likely to now be available in ways that facilitate life satisfaction and pleasure (Osborne, 2012).

In the paragraphs that follow, each of these three tasks will be detailed.

The challenge of preserving and maintaining one's identity and self-worth

When people end their paid employment, they also end their identification with the role or category title that they have been associated with as a paid worker. As a result, they have to deal with the loss of an often major piece of their identity, typically a main way that they have viewed themselves to create a definition of who they are and who they have been (Erikson, 1963; Feldman, 1994). Especially in the period right after retirement, people also have to deal with the unfamiliarity of everyday events and as a result, with a life that is less familiar, predictable, and continuous with their past. Given, as noted, that people tend to retire relatively late-in-life age, they may also simultaneously have to contend with concurrent "inner" physical changes associated with aging that may add to the challenge of coping with the outer changes that are occurring (Atchley, 1993).

Because not everyone takes pride in their work role, or identifies with their work, several factors are likely to determine how much a person's self-worth is affected when they give up the "identity designators" that people usually attached to work. These factors include: the importance and value that the person has associated to the role and titles that they have retired from; the centrality of these roles and titles in the overall way that the person defines themselves; and lastly, their perception of the nature and degree of changes in ways that others see and relate to them once they are no longer "workers". For example, a person's identity and self-esteem are likely to be relatively lower if after retiring they believe that others now view them as "aged" or less capable (Ekerdt & DeViney, 1990; Wang, Henkens, & van Solinge, 2011).

Several other factors may also cause a person to feel self-critical and experience a diminished sense of self-worth after retirement. They may, for example, castigate themselves for no longer producing income and as a result, being less able to contribute financially to the well-being of their family, or they may compare themselves to their former "working self" or others who continue to work, and view themselves as a lazy or unproductive person (Atchley, 1993). Self-criticism following retirement is especially likely if a person has been told from an early age that it is virtuous to be busy and bad to "sit around". For example, many people have been graded in elementary school on the degree to which they displayed such "good" character traits as effort, industriousness, and efficient time use. As a result they may feel guilty when they are not required to do something productive or useful and instead choose to do what they want and enjoy doing.

Further, after retirement, even if a person does desire to engage in a productive activity, a person may have difficulty in identifying just what this activity would be since they can no longer rely on the main former criterion that they are likely to have used in the past – their paid work. Contrary to the field of economics where there is a formal definition of productivity (i.e. any activity that results in a product that has added to the stock and flow of valued goods and services traded in the market place) (Syverson, 2011), when people leave the "market place", they have to rely on subjective indicators and the opinion of others to judge if they are using their time productively.

Cultural beliefs about wellness may also influence how self-critical and how pressured a person feels to be busy and use their time well. Most people are likely to have repeatedly heard that to ward off both illness and the rate of physical decline, they need to be active. Thus, they are likely to feel self-critical and worried if, following retirement, they are not as "lively" as they or others think they ought to be.

The challenge of creating a life structure and allocating increased discretionary time

In the period following retirement people may have the largest amount of discretionary time – time without required tasks, since their early school days. As a result, allocating this increased amount of discretionary time can be difficult and disorienting, especially since now, without work obligations, people have a much greater role in selecting the activities that they wish to engage in and the amount of time that they wish to devote to each of the activities that they select (Atchley, 1989; Osborne, 2012). Adding to this challenge are changes not only in what they do but also in regard to what they are no longer required to do. For example, they no longer are required to get up at the same time as they did in the past, travel in the same way that they did to get to work, or go to a particular grocery to get their morning coffee.

In general most people cope with these life changes by focusing either on life goals that are familiar to them and continuous with the goals that they have valued and maintained in the past, or by focusing on wishes that they intended to fulfill "when they have the time". These latter, wished-for goals, often include an element of novelty and a desire to create a new chapter in the "story" of their life. Whether a person selects familiar or novel goals, however, the act of setting a goal itself, of having a future target that the person can expend effort towards following retirement is found to lessen a person's sense of disorientation and uncertainty and enhance their well-being (Hershey, Jacobs-Lawson, & Neukam, 2002).

In formal surveys, the most frequently reported goals and fantasies mentioned by retirees soon after retirement include: travelling to a new, previously imagined setting; moving or buying a new or second residence, often in a nature-like setting such as by a lake; acquiring knowledge about something that either was previously unfamiliar, or was of interest in the past but never explored (e.g., taking specialized classes, making "site" visits to unfamiliar, exotic places); engaging in an activity that involves creative expression (e.g., learning to paint or play a musical instrument); and lastly, participating in an altruistic activity. An underlying theme present in all these goals and fantasies seems to be a wish to have new and unfamiliar experiences – to feel like an explorer engaged in an adventure that will result in personal growth (Gupta & Hershey, 2016).

The importance of personal growth

Thus, people may feel a conflict after retirement. On the one hand, they may believe there is a benefit, at least at first, to keeping to the familiar, yet on the other hand, they often desire to experience something new. As a result, they may feel stressed as they try to decide how much of their familiar experiences and routines they should maintain and when, how, and to what degree they should seek novelty and unfamiliarity.

In general, people's well-being is found to be relatively higher in the period following retirement if they do both – if they attempt to keep to familiar roles and activities that help them maintain their identity and foster a sense of predictability while simultaneously, as indicated by the survey that was just described, plan and begin to experiment with ways that they may experience novelty and anticipate an adventure (Maslow, 1971; McCrea, 1992; Baltes, 1999).

What is also found is that whether using past, familiar experiences or exploring new areas, people are likely to achieve a relatively higher sense of well-being and life satisfaction following retirement if they attempt to enlarge their knowledge, abilities, and emotional repertoire. Thus when people engage in hobbies, projects, and other learning activities that they find stimulating and foster curiosity, they are less anxious and believe that they will maintain their current level of cognitive and physical functioning and slow their rate of biological decline (Butrica & Schaner, 2005; Gregory, Nettlebeck, & Wilson, 2010).

The following vignette illustrates several of the key ideas noted in the selective review of the literature:

Martin, aged 68, had been thinking about retirement since he turned 65. A professor in a graduate program at a university, he couldn't come to a clear decision. He would think, on the one hand, how repetitive his life had become – how he got up at the same time each day, traveled the same roads, got coffee at the same place and time, and how annoyed he was at the politics where he worked – the incessant demand for budget cuts and increased productivity. Yet, on the other hand, he still got a tremendous amount of pleasure when he noticed the admiring look of his students, was inspired when he interacted with a student who was highly inquisitive and engaged, and liked having a regular income and not having to figure out how long his savings needed to last.

The department chairman asked to meet with Martin. At the meeting he told Martin that because of cuts in the university budget, Martin would need to teach an undergraduate class, something he had not done since the very beginning of his teaching career, in addition to his regular graduate teaching responsibilities. Usually a cautious person, Martin impulsively said no. He told the chairman that instead of agreeing to the request, he would resign at the end of the semester. Sitting in his office afterwards, Martin felt both relieved that he had finally made a choice, yet anxious as he considered the unknowns that lay ahead. He tried to picture a life without such familiar demands as preparing lectures, teaching, or meeting with colleagues, and especially, without his professor title which he was especially proud of and had almost always elicited respect from others.

During the three months left in the semester, Martin continued to feel sure that the choice to retire was the right one but wasn't sure how he would fill his time when he stopped working. Since graduating and receiving his doctorate 37 years ago, Martin had worked about 60 hours a week. And when he did have "down time", he always felt that he had to do something productive and never was able to simply sit still.

With the semester over, instead of being his usual structured self, Martin thought that he would be spontaneous. He would start each day without a "to do list" and decide what he would do based on what "emerged" during the day. After a few days of trying this approach, he realized it was not working. As yet, he did not have an epiphany during the day that let him know what he should do, and so far, he mostly felt unanchored and bored. He decided that he needed to be his usual self. So at the start of each day, Martin made a plan by sitting, being self-reflective, and noting what he was thinking and feeling and then tried to use his thoughts and feelings to decide what he would do.

Martin also realized that without his university ID, he not only now felt "ordinary" but also, at times self-conscious when around others, for example, when shopping at the supermarket, he felt embarrassed, as if others were viewing him as a lazy person – as someone who should be working but wasn't.

Part two: Strategies to manage the challenges that arise in relation to retirement

The following ideas and strategies can be used by clinicians if a person raises one or more of the following concerns during a clinical encounter.

The idea of a "bridge" or transition to full retirement

When a person is unsure of their readiness to retire, or especially when they have been forced to retire involuntarily, a clinician can describe the increasingly popular idea of bridge employment. Instead of fully retiring, the clinician explains, many people either choose to gradually phase out of their career job or engage in new work activities, often on a part-time basis. By doing so, the clinician can explain that the person is more likely to acquire additional financial and social resources, reduce stress, and maintain a sense of purpose, feelings of productivity, and continuity with their past experiences. As a result, they "smooth" the transition from working to not working.

Further, by retiring in phases, a person is able to try out having more discretionary time and experiment with ways to fill this time. In addition, they can also try out new roles, pursue existing or new leisure activities, and incrementally adjust to the likely decrease in structure and increase in choice that they now have available in regard to how they want to spend their time (Davies & Cartwright, 2011; Sewdas et al., 2017).

The clinician can also point out that empirically people who choose to gradually transition from work to non-work are relatively more likely to maintain their preretirement levels of life satisfaction during the retirement transition compared to retirees who do not engage in bridge employment (Dingemans, 2012).

Managing discretionary time

When talking to someone who has just retired, the clinician can help a person adapt to the alterations in life roles and questions about how to allocate time by suggesting that the person consider establishing a tentative life structure that includes at least some of their past routines and activities, particularly over the next few months. By maintaining a sense of sameness, the person is likely to lessen feelings of instability and unpredictability that most people feel during periods of significant change and more likely to increase feelings of control and orderliness. Further, by establishing and maintaining a structure and routines, the person is giving themselves time to adapt to retirement and thoughtfully explore, reflect, and carefully shape the structure and content of how they want the next phase of their life to be.

The clinician might also mention that as paid work ends and the person has more choice as to how they want to spend their time, many people find it helpful to ask themselves several deep and complicated questions such as: What do I see as my main purpose(s) or reasons for wanting to live? What do I most value? What do I want to accomplish while I am still able to influence the outcomes that are most important to me? What do I want to now do with the likely increased amount of discretionary time that I now have available to experience pleasure and satisfaction? And lastly, how do I intend to balance my own interests with the demands on time that others now may make (Van Tilburg & Igou, 2012)?

The clinician can suggest that the person could use the answers to these questions in several ways. He or she might brainstorm and consider all the things that he or she could do and then thoughtfully identify activities and times that they might want to commit to each activity. By doing so, the person is considering what most matters to them, typically based on the degree of pleasure and satisfaction that they have experienced in the past. The person could then try out a plan for a defined period of time (e.g. one month), and based on the "try out", evaluate if they are satisfied with the structure that they have created. If they are, they are likely to continue to maintain it; if they conclude that they are unsatisfied, they could make revisions and continue to "investigate".

Instead of this highly methodical and carefully thought out plan, the clinician could point out another option that many people employ. They could improvise – try a variety of things while being self-aware and self-reflective, keep track of what seems most fulfilling, and continuously apportion and adjust the discretionary time that they available in an on-going, spontaneous manner, based on the pleasure and satisfaction they are getting from their day-to-day experiences. Finally, the clinician can suggest what many would consider the most sensible alternative, to combine the two strategies. The person might develop a general outline of what they think matters most to them, fill in and organize their discretionary time based on these activities, and then improvise while being open to new experiences, and continuously adjust their choices based on what they learn and experience (Smith, Wagaman, & Handley, 2009).

Managing the increased risk of boredom

One risk of having a greater amount of discretionary time which the clinician can mention is boredom (Voldanovich & Watt, 1999). The clinician can explain that with less of a need to fill time in a required, externally-imposed way, a person may occasionally be at a loss as to what to do to feel engaged and experience pleasure or satisfaction. As a result, the person may feel restless and unable to concentrate. While boredom is an aversive state, the clinician can point out that it can also be beneficial. It provides an important signal – an indication of a need to exert more effort to identify experiences that are interesting and involving (Elpidorou, 2014).

Because boredom is frequently triggered by familiarity and repetitiveness, the clinician can explain that when the person receives this "signal", that makes salient the fact that they are bored, they might seek and try to engage in activities that are unfamiliar to them relative to the activities that they have previously engaged in; make sure that whatever activities they select include variety, either in regard to the content of the activity or the manner in which it is carried out; and that the activity chosen is complex – it requires a relatively higher level of concentration to perform adequately (Eastwood, Frischen, Fenske, & Smilek, 2012).

Managing the identity and self-worth challenges that may be triggered by retirement

Not only is a person's identity or sense of sameness threatened by changes in the ways that a person uses time after retirement, but as noted, it is also threatened by the loss of the key roles that they have used in the past to define who they are. To help a person maintain their sense of identity, the clinician can explain that it is helpful for a person to focus on who they continue to be rather than on who they no longer are (Atchley, 1993), and especially to focus on the "non-paid work aspects" of their identity, that is, the roles that they continue to enact and experience as meaningful and desirable (e.g. the roles of a loving father, a good friend, a good son) (Wang, Henkens, and van Solinge, 2011).

The clinician can also explain that still another way they can remain focused on what is stable and enduring about them is to be aware of the values and standards that they have consistently used in the past to make choices – their core beliefs as to the kind of person that they want and feel they ought to be. By being aware of how they are consistently keeping to their "guiding principles", the clinician can point out that in essential ways, they are and continue to be the same person that they were in the past.

During this discussion, the clinician can mention that some people after retiring feel a decline in self-worth. They may no longer feel "productive", and may doubt they have sufficient value or that others may view them as having less value. To counter these doubts and highlight what they feel they still can provide is valuable, the clinician can point out that some people, for example, put more effort into supporting family members, volunteer, or counsel a mentee in an area in which they have accumulated a high level of expertise (Weinstein, Xie, & Cleanthous, 1995). The clinician can note that when people choose to engage in these types of "other-directed" activities they often need to decide how much time they want to devote to them out of the total amount of time they have available (Anderson, 2007).

When addressing the issues of identity and self-worth, the clinician might reiterate the need to ensure that the person is spending a sufficient amount of time with people he or she cares about. The clinician can emphasize that it is through contact with long-standing friends and family members that a person is likely to gain the type of feedback that they need to feel they are still who they were, still matter, and still have value (Froidevaux, Hirschi, & Wang, 2016). Finally, the clinician can point out that people are found to have relatively higher levels of well-being if they include physical activity in the time that they have available and make sure that they get sufficient sleep (Olds et al., 2018).

Maintaining and enhancing vitality and personal growth

Similar to when the clinician may have described the typical goals and fantasies that most people have when they retire, the clinician can highlight the benefit of viewing retirement as the start of a new chapter and not the start of a final one. Towards this end, the clinician can encourage the person to try to be open to engaging in experiences that are novel, particularly experiences that differ from the experiences that they engaged in while working (Csikszentmihalyi, 1975). The clinician can describe choices other people have made when they have tried to create a new chapter. These choices have included: volunteering and performing unfamiliar tasks in an unfamiliar setting, ideally for a group of people that the person has little prior exposure to (e.g. a food bank in an impoverished, multi-cultural neighborhood); engaging in a hobby that draws on skills that they have not utilized before (e.g. playing a musical instrument); or participating in an activity that the person may have considered in the past but never actually attempted, either due to a lack of available time or anxiety.

The clinician might also mention that some people choose to engage in an activity that they had enjoyed in the past but had not done for many years, such as travelling to a place that they travelled to when they were young, or restarting a hobby that gave them a great deal of pleasure in the past. Finally, the clinician can mention that some people use the increased discretionary time that they now have available to deal with regrets – to do things they feel they should have done in the past but never did.

Once a person identifies an opportunity to either attempt to have a novel experience or to do something they have not done for a very long time, the clinician should mention that they may be tempted to procrastinate. The clinician can explain that it is normal to feel anxious when considering the prospect of "stepping into" the unfamiliar (Baltes, 1999) and that in order to lessen the hesitation that they may feel, it is helpful to focus on the hoped-for payoffs that they anticipate they may experience once they actually do what they are considering; to focus, for example, on the pleasure and satisfaction that they will feel from learning a new subject, or the reassurance that they will gain from still feeling vital and capable (Kasden, 2009).

Further, to maximize the benefits of engaging in novel experiences, the clinician might emphasize that after completing such an experience, it is important for the person to make time available to reflect on what has been felt and thought. In this way the person is more likely to be able to be aware of and label what they found valuable, and by doing so, more likely to be clearer going forward as to what is likely to make them happy and satisfied (McCrae, 1992; Brown & Ryan, 2003; Stephan, 2009).

The following vignette illustrates several of the ideas and strategies that have been mentioned:

Martin's annual medical check-up was scheduled for the week after his official last day at work. When the doctor asked what had changed since the last visit, Martin said what had been most momentous was that he was no longer a worker, something that he had been since he was 14. He told the doctor about his feeling of disorientation, his generally overcautious life style, his overly strong work ethic, and especially, his confusion as to whether to just be himself or push himself to be different than his usual self.

The doctor briefly described what he knew of the literature about health and retirement, emphasizing the importance of being active and maintaining routines, while at the same time, seeking growth opportunities. The doctor went on to mention that many of his patients expected their life to be dramatically different following retirement, and yet when he saw them subsequently, in many ways even without work, they said that most things seemed relatively the same.

Now, about six months after retiring and his discussion with his physician, Martin realized, like the physician had said, he continued to be who he was – a person who needed to keep to routines yet also a person who wanted to push himself, at least occasionally, to leave his "comfort zone". Thus, as he had done his entire professional life, Martin got up at the same, very early time each day, researched an academic topic, and wrote for about an hour. Yet, with great trepidation, he also decided to give in to his wife's long-standing wish to take a long flight to Europe, a flight that he had always envisioned as an invitation, once on the plane, to feel trapped, claustrophobic, and possibly have a panic attack.

Martin also came to realize that he was still who he had always been. Although several books that he had read about retirement suggested meditation, he was unable to sit still for long periods of time. In the language of these books, he could see that he was not the type to stay focused on the "now". Instead, he knew that he was a perpetually restless person who was driven to not waste time and always be doing something that he felt was meaningful. But, as the doctor had said, he also knew that he needed to feel that he could still learn and grow and in this way avoid the anxiety-producing thought that, figuratively and literally, he was shrinking.

Thus, to try something different and in keeping with his interest before becoming an academic of becoming a legal aid attorney, Martin decided to take a seminar on poverty and justice at a local university. During the seminar, the teacher mentioned that a newly formed prison release program was seeking volunteers to be teacher-mentors. Martin volunteered. Almost immediately, even though he was working with very different students than he had in the past, he realized how much he still enjoyed being a teacher and how engaging it was to listen to the very different life experiences of these just-released mentees.

Although Martin felt that by taking a class and volunteering he had created a reasonably satisfying routine, something still felt missing. He had kept in touch with several colleagues who had also retired about the same time that he had and were now either in the process of selling their homes and moving, or had already done so. When he listened to the changes that they were experiencing, to the new chapter they had inserted between their previous chapter and the terrifying "end chapter" that he had trouble keeping out of his mind, Martin was envious. He tried to consider what might be an exciting or pleasurable next phase of life for him, but at least for now, he was at a loss.

Summary

Retirement is likely to result in major alterations in a person's roles, relationships, daily routines, self-view, and beliefs about how they are viewed by others. As a consequence, retirement has the potential to bring about a high level of stress as well as opportunities for growth. In order to maintain a sense of continuity, predictability, and control, especially in the period immediately following retirement, it is important that a person establish and maintain a tentative life structure and set of routines.

Since a person's work role is often a key element of their identity and self-worth, after a person retires, a clinician can help the person clarify what they now believe are the central attributes that define them and to focus on who they still are rather than who they no longer are or can be. In addition, the clinician can help the person thoughtfully address how they want to use the increased discretionary time that is now likely to be available.

The clinician can also encourage a person to be self-reflective and carefully consider how they want to allocate their time and select activities that are stimulating and engaging. Finally, the clinician can mention the risk of boredom and a major antidote – identifying and pursuing experiences that are engaging and likely to result in personal growth.

Chapter 4

A second major challenge to a person's well-being as they age

The increasing number of deaths of significant others

Part one: A selective review of the literature

Overview

The experience of loss becomes an increasingly common event the longer a person lives (de Vries & Johnson, 2002), as is the feeling of being a survivor who has outlived many of the individuals in their friendship and family social networks (Forster, Stein, Lobner, Pabst et al., 2018). The oldest-old are found to complain that they are one of the few left among the people they have known (de Vries & Johnson, 2002).

The types of losses that people experience as they age tend to occur in a fairly typical sequence. First, people who are older than the person, such as parents, aunts, and uncles, are likely to die; then, people who are close to the person's own age, such as spouses, siblings and life-long friends are likely to die. And, finally, if the person reaches old-old age, people who are younger than the person, such as the person's children, are likely to die (d'Epinay, Cavalli, & Guillet, 2009–2010).

When the losses of significant others accrue, in addition to sorrow, people are also likely to feel unanchored – to feel they are losing their history, the main links that they have had to their past, as well as the ability to share events and memories with others. Their social network is likely to shrink in size and become more restricted. As a result, without the recognition from people who have truly known them, they are more likely to feel depressed, in part because they have lost a central means of clarifying, confirming, and correcting self-perceptions (de Vries & Johnson, 2002) and affirming who they are and have been (Forster et al., 2018).

In addition, when people lose their friends and family members, their confidantes or "secure base" (Bowlby, 1982), they are likely to feel profoundly alone. They are without the people who have been sensitive and responsive to their needs and who have supplied them with concrete assistance, comfort, and reassurance when they were upset (Edward, 2016). Especially in the period following these types of losses, therefore, people are likely to feel unsafe, tend to withdraw and are less willing to explore new possibilities or take risks (Bowlby, 1980).

A person's self-esteem is also likely to be affected. When a person's spouse, close friend, or sibling dies, the person tends to lose a primary source of feedback – of appreciation and validation – data that they are likely to have used to feel that they have mattered, been worthy, and valuable (Connidis & Davies, 1990; Edward, 2016).

Finally, the person is likely to experience an increased level of anxiety about death, especially if the people who have died were close to their own age. Using these close others who died as a "yardstick" to compare when events in their own life will occur, as a way of foretelling their own future, they are more likely to think about their own mortality (de Vries & Johnson, 2002), feel that their death is closer in time, and that they have only a limited amount of control in delaying this eventuality (Becker, 1973; Connidis & Davies, 1990; Roberto & Stanis, 1994).

In the paragraphs that follow, each of the major types of losses people are likely to experience as they age will be detailed, along with the effect of these losses on their sense of well-being.

The loss of a spouse

As noted, the death of a spouse most frequently occurs in young-old rather than old-old age (d'Epinay, Cavalli, & Spini, 2003). Women in old-old age are much more likely than men to lose a spouse, primarily because women tend to be younger than the men they marry (Bennett & Soulsby, 2012). Thus, approximately two thirds of women over the age of 75 have lost their spouse compared to only one quarter of men (Lopata, 1996).

The loss of a spouse often affects almost every domain of a person's life. As a result, especially in the year following bereavement, a person's sense of well-being is likely to significantly decline. A person's spouse is typically their primary companion, and after his or her death, the person is likely to feel a painful sense of being "without" and as a result, experience many symptoms of both grief and depression (d'Epinay et al., 2009–2010).

In addition, the person is likely to feel uncertain about how to fill his or her time, and specifically, about who to tell about everyday events (Connidis & Davies, 1990). The risk of loneliness therefore is especially high, particularly if the person's spouse was responsible for determining the size and composition of their social network (Dykstra & de Jong Gierveld, 2004; Spahni, Bennett, & Perrig-Chiello, 2015).

The loss of close friends

The death of close friends in later life is a regular occurrence. For example, in one study about one third of people over the age of 65 and one half of people over the age of 85 lost a close friend through death each year (de Vries & Johnson, 2002). Even though quite common, the literature on the loss of close friends late in life is sparse. Based on the few studies that are available, when a close friend dies people tend to experience a profound sense of emptiness similar to the type of emptiness that they feel when a family member dies (Sklar & Hartley, 1990).

While the meaning attached to the term "close friend" can vary, in the present context, the term is used to describe a long-term, reciprocal relationship with someone who has been both a confidante and a companion, as well as a repository of shared, cherished memories. Relationships with close friends therefore can have a strong, often more positive influence on a person's sense of well-being than relationships with family members, as suggested by the finding that after the loss of a spouse, people turn to their close friends more frequently than family members for support and companionship (Roberto & Stanis, 1994).

There are differences between men and women in the nature of their close friend relationships. Women, compared to men, are found to value the personal, emotional, and affectionate elements of a close relationship and as a result, are more likely to share confidential information with their close friends. Men, on the other hand, are found to value sharing activities and mutual interests with close friends and, as a consequence, are less likely to disclose intimate information with their close friends (Roberto & Stanis, 1994). Thus, while women tend to have people outside their marriage that they share their most private thoughts with, men tend to use their wives as confidantes. The result is that when their often sole confidante dies, men are especially likely to feel lonely and bereft (Strain & Chappell, 1982).

Compared to coping with other losses as people age, coping with the loss of a close friend is particularly challenging. This type of loss is not usually recognized in an organized or ritualized way so that, in contrast to being called a widow or orphan, for example, there are no titles to describe the loss of a friend (de Vries & Johnson, 2002). As a result, people are less likely to receive the support that they tend to get, for instance, when a family member dies. In addition, given the likelihood of having had frequent contact with the close friend who died, the person is likely to feel lonely and more socially isolated afterward, especially if their social network has already shrunk a great deal (Roberto & Stanis, 1994).

The loss of a parent

As mentioned, the death of a parent most frequently occurs in young-old rather than old-old age (d'Epinay, Cavalli, & Spini, 2003). Since it is considered by most an expectable loss, a loss in keeping with what is thought of as the natural order of life events, it tends to be relatively less disruptive and has less impact on a person's well-being. In addition to the effect of expectations, this type of loss may also be relatively less disruptive because as people age their parents are less likely to have served as primary caregivers and attachment figures to the same degree as they did in the past. Thus, a person is likely to have turned less to them for support and more likely to have relied on spouses, close friends, and off-spring (d'Epinay et al., 2003; Marks, Jun, & Song, 2007).

Further, usually starting when people are in their early sixties, they are more likely to provide support to their parents than receive support from them (Marks et al., 2007). As a result, in addition to feelings of distress, people may also experience a sense of relief – an end to a period of uncertainty and stress and a lifting of the burden of being in a caretaking role, often while managing their usual, everyday responsibilities (Rostila & Saarela, 2011).

The loss of a sibling

When a person's siblings die, compared to other types of losses, the person is likely to feel that they have lost a primary means of sharing and validating their memories, especially their memories of early life events (Moss & Moss, 1989). Depending on the degree of closeness that has existed between themselves and their siblings, a person may also feel that they have lost a confidante and a key element of their functional support system (Connidis & Davies, 1990; d'Epinay et al., 2009–2010).

The loss of an adult child

Unlike the loss of a parent when people are older, the loss of an adult child is often experienced as a violation of the expected, natural order. As a result, it is likely to have a profound, markedly adverse effect on a person's well-being. After the loss of an adult child, a person is likely to become depressed, have survivor's guilt, and typically wish that they had died instead of their child (Moss, Lesher, & Moss, 1986–1987; d'Epinay et al., 2009–2010).

Especially in the period following the death of an adult child, people are likely to become isolated, anxious, and insecure, at times, because in old age their adult child may have been their primary source of instrumental support (Ward, LaGory, & Sherman, 1982). Thus, following the death of an adult child, people are more likely to experience an increase in health problems, have difficulty identifying a life purpose, and difficulty in viewing life as worth living (Arbuckle & de Vries, 1995).

The factors that influence the nature and degree of people's reactions to loss

As would be expected, people vary in the way they react to loss and the degree to which they react. The factors that are likely to influence the impact of a particular loss on an individual's well-being include the degree to which they were close and had seen or spoken to the person frequently; felt "clarity" rather than ambivalence towards the person; depended on the person to meet important needs; and were forewarned that the loss was imminent. In addition, people are likely to be more negatively impacted by a loss if, at the time of the loss, they were experiencing a high level of stress, their coping capacity was depleted, and they had inadequate social support (Wortman & Silver, 1990).

Further, as the number of losses the person experiences accumulate – as more and more people with whom they have had a significant relationship die, as would be expected – they are less likely to be able to maintain a state of well-being. They may feel like an "orphan", and as mentioned at the beginning of the chapter, with few living others who truly know them and who they truly know, are less able to share everyday events and concerns, talk to others who remember what they remember, and who are aware and participated in the important occasions that they have experienced. As a result, they are at increased risk of losing their motivation to socialize and make new friends (Rook, 2009), and with a decreased sense of connection to others, at increased risk of feeling empty and forlorn (Weiss, 1973; de Jong Gierveld & Havens, 2004).

Thus, as these losses accumulate, in addition to the decrease in instrumental or practical assistance and support that is likely to occur, as noted, people are also less likely to feel embedded in a social network (Forster et al., 2018). As a result, they tend to have less opportunity to engage in activities that they perceive as meaningful to "fill their day" and are more likely to experience a sense of instability. Without a "safety net" therefore, they are likely to feel increasingly stressed and vulnerable and believe that more unpleasant, uncontrollable events are coming at a time when they have less social support to buffer and deal with these events (Marks et al., 2007; Forster et al., 2018).

The following vignette illustrates several of the key ideas noted in the selective review of the literature:

Sitting at the kitchen table after getting home from the funeral, Sarah, age 87, tried to find words to capture what she was feeling. The closest that she could come up with was "survivor". With the death of her best friend, Clara, a person she had known since she was a little girl, there were no "others" who were still alive and who truly knew her, who she had shared all the ups and downs with – all the moments that had mattered; who understood just what she meant when she made references to words and people from the past; who understood her personal jokes, or why something had special significance to her. Nostalgic, she reviewed all the people who had "disappeared" – first her mother at age 8; then her father when she was in her twenties; followed by her older sister, three years ago, and then Sol, her husband, last year.

Slumped in the chair, forlorn and lonely, she felt as if she had just lost the last remaining keeper of her history and identity, the person that she had she spoken to everyday; who listened attentively both to important and trivial things, and the person that she cared about and who she knew cared about her. They were no longer the two mutually supportive buddies, each making the other feel valued. While her daughter Amy grudgingly checked on her periodically, it always seemed like a chore; when visiting or on the phone, Amy had little to say and acted as if she was fulfilling an obligation that she seemed to get little personal benefit from.

Crying, Sarah thought of another word that fit how she was feeling – "without" – as she considered the empty days ahead and the likelihood of her own not too distant death. Unlike past times when she thought about dying, however, she now felt relief rather than fear.

Part two: Coping with the challenge of accumulating loss in later life

The following ideas and strategies can be used by clinicians if a person raises one or more of the following concerns during a clinical encounter.

Helping the person maintain a balanced focus

When talking to a person attempting to cope with the yearning and ache of loneliness after the death of a person they have been close to, the clinician can encourage the person to focus not only on what they miss about the relationship but also focus on what they have valued and are grateful for. For example, the clinician can explain that the person might review moments that are especially memorable and while doing so, try to visualize and label the specific ingredients that composed these precious moments (e.g. being hugged, the sound of her laugh, his enthusiasm). The clinician can suggest that the person might consider the bond that they have had with the person and what about that bond seems special (e.g. it represented a commitment to acknowledge how important each person was to the other; it represented loyalty).

The clinician might also suggest that the person try to identify a positive life lesson or legacy they derived from the relationship – a lesson that they can use and value going forward (e.g. that even when someone is very ill, they can be loving and relatively selfless). Finally, the clinician could point out that by emulating and attempting to match the actions of the people they miss, they can maintain a "continuing bond" with them and, in a sense, keep them forever alive (Klass, Silverman, & Nickman, 1996).

Enhancing the motivation to live

If a person has experienced multiple losses in a relatively short time, they may feel unanchored and without their "social convoy" (i.e. the people who they have travelled with over a long period of time whose presence provides a sense of security). As a result, they may lose their will to live. To counterbalance the risk of despair, a clinician can suggest that the person first reexamine and clarify their belief system – the values and principles that they have relied on in the past in order to identify what matters most to them (e.g. god, their children) – and based on this reassessment, see if they can find aspects of their life that might still provide them with a reason to stay alive.

Since many people may not be able to identify a set of compelling reasons on their own, the clinician might encourage the person to consider an established system of beliefs to identify a set of meaningful goals that they can use to regain their sense of purpose, in keeping with the empirical finding that as people get older, ascribing to a religion tends to facilitate well-being (Baumeister, 1991). Since strong atheistic beliefs facilitate coping as much as strong religious beliefs, the clinician can point out that the content of the belief system is less important than the strength of their beliefs, and highlight that by having a belief system they can gain an explanation that could help them accept the losses that have occurred. The clinician can also mention that the person might consider joining a group with others who share these beliefs (e.g. a church or synagogue) and in this way possibly gain support and comfort (Wilkinson & Coleman, 2010).

Clarifying life goals and challenging the risk of social isolation

If the person continues to have difficulty identifying or reestablishing a sense of purpose, as the fog of grief begins to lift, the clinician can suggest that the person might review goals that in the past have provided them with the feeling that their life had meaning and value. Based on this review, the clinician can explain, the person could consider how they might wish to allocate their time now.

If enacting these former goals involved the family and friends who have died, the clinician can point out that the person might consider if there are still aspects of what they had done that they now can continue to do on their own, or if they are ready and willing to be open to novelty and being social, they could look for new opportunities.

The clinician can highlight that it is most important to not withdraw; that by remaining active, the person is more likely to reduce feelings of loneliness and the sense that their social world is shrinking.

Acceptance

As has been mentioned in relation to many other issues that arise and impact a person's well-being as they age, the clinician can explain that the painful loss of a close relationship is one more instance in which a person has to work at accepting what they cannot change. Towards this end the clinician can say that many people cope by trying to view death as something neither to fear or welcome but instead as an unalterable given.

The clinician can also point out, as described in Chapter 1, that people are likely to be less anxious about death if they are able to develop a conception of death that is either positive (e.g. that a person will enter an idyllic afterlife) or at least less terrifying (e.g. a person will return to the state that existed prior to their birth); and if they can, going forward, seek, affirm, and savor experiences that they do find meaningful and valuable (Wong & Tomer, 2011).

The following vignette illustrates several of the strategies that have been mentioned:

It was about six months since she attended the funeral and Sarah was increasingly withdrawn, isolated, and sad. She felt angry, abandoned by those she had counted on, and at times did not speak to anyone for days at a time. She increasingly felt unanchored, as if she were a tiny speck floating in a large space. As had always been her routine, she was up very early one morning when the phone rang. To her surprise it was her daughter Amy, who said that she wanted to come over and talk. Sarah had been feeling especially hurt by Amy's lack of concern and her failure to "pay Sarah back" for all the sacrifices that she felt she had made as a parent as Amy was growing up.

Sitting at the kitchen table, Amy told her mother that she had made an appointment for the two of them to meet with a geriatric social worker the next day. Amy said that she had gotten the woman's name from a friend who said that the social worker was an expert in problems of older people and their families and had helped her friend and her friend's mother. Amy said she was worried about Sarah because of how angry and bitter she always seemed to be. She told her mother that she complained constantly and as a result, most people did not want to call or visit.

During the appointment with the social worker, Amy told her mother for the first time how hurt she had been that her mother never acknowledged how awful it was for her when her marriage was ending. She said that Sarah had never offered any help or support, yet now expected her to be kind and attentive. At first Sarah protested but with the social worker's help, saw her daughter's point of view and apologized. She explained that while Amy was going through her divorce, her own mother was at the end of her life and that she was very drained.

The social worker pointed out that Sarah and Amy seemed to care a great deal about each other and to want to be close. The social worker suggested that they pick a specific day each week when they would meet and make a ritual – a regularly occurring time when they could share what was important to each of them.

The social worker then turned to Sarah and said that when Amy set up the appointment she mentioned that one of Sarah's closest friends had died. She wondered if Sarah was having a tough time coping with the loss. Sarah acknowledged that she was; she felt very isolated, angry, probably self-pitying, and lately, especially alone and unhappy.

The social worker suggested that since she had become so isolated that she, perhaps with Amy's help, might want to try to find things to do with other people so that she could feel less alone. And instead of looking only at what was now missing from her life, she might consider, when she woke up each day, what she had experienced the day before that she felt was positive and she appreciated. The social worker explained that by focusing more on what was okay, Sarah might be less sad and negative. Lastly, she suggested that Sarah might try to be more aware of when she was angry and complaining when talking with others, and if she wanted, when they next met, she could help her clarify why she was so angry. Together they could then try to come up with alternative, more adaptive ways of acting at these times.

On the way home from the appointment, Amy told Sarah that a new Rabbi had been hired at the local synagogue and had started a seniors' program. Amy said that she would call and find out the day and time of the next senior activity. She gave the information to Sarah who, with a great deal of trepidation, attended the event. When Amy called to see how the experience was, Sarah said it was good to be active and be around other people but strange to not know anyone, and at her age, to feel that she was back in grade school, at the start of the school year, awkwardly trying to meet new people.

Summary

As people age, the loss of people that they have been close to is likely to be an increasingly frequent and highly stressful event. When more and more of the people they have known die, a person is likely to have difficulty holding on to the shared memories that have allowed them to view their lives as familiar and continuous with their past. Further, as more and more of their "social convoy" die, a person is likely to feel unsafe and lonely, and without these often life-long companions and confidantes, to feel socially isolated. In addition, the reminders of the inevitability of death are also likely to cause the person to feel increasingly anxious about their own mortality.

The types of losses that people tend to experience as they age include spouses, close friends, their biological family, and if they live until they are very old, adult children. While a person, of course, can lose someone who matters to them at any age, typically people lose their parents first, in young-old age, and their adult children last, in old-old age. The effects of a particular loss on a person's well-being vary and depend in part on the degree to which the person felt close to the individual who died, and the degree to which they have depended on that individual to fulfill important needs.

If the number of losses a person experiences increase to the point that there are very few people left who the person feels close to, the person may feel like an orphan, an individual who lacks others who know them and who they know. They are also more likely to feel that they are on their own, without others to spend time with, and others who will support them when they need assistance.

To cope with these losses, a clinician can help the person balance their focus. Instead of being preoccupied exclusively with the aspects of the relationships that they miss, the clinician can help the person focus on and savor the aspects of the relationships that they have found to be precious. Even though a person may be grieving and still primarily focus on what they have lost, the clinician can note that generally, over time, people are able to look forward and identify a belief system or source of meaning that provides them with a rationale to stay engaged and live rather than withdraw. The clinician can also point out that if the person finds a belief system, or develops a personal sense of what now most matters to them, it can motivate them to seek new experiences.

Chapter 5

Aging, well-being, and life-regrets

Part one: A selective review of the literature

Overview

To reminisce as people reach old age – to look back, review life choices, and understand how a person has arrived at the place in life that they now occupy – is a common occurrence. In particular, when people review their past choices, they are likely to focus on times when they faced a conflict between two courses of action and had to decide either to do something that was tempting but risky, or not do something that they later wished they had done, but at the time, had found too frightening (Butler, 1963).

Can people reach old age without regrets?

Thus, as people enter old age, they are likely to reconsider their life accomplishments and failures, continuously construct and revise versions of their life history, often using changing perspectives of the past and incorporating new experiences, and think about the decreasing opportunity that they will have to undo or fulfill whatever they have regretted (Timmer, Westerhof, & Dittman-Kohli, 2005). Given the number of important choices that people make during the course of their lifetime, it is not surprising that up to 90% of people feel that they should have done some things differently than they did and report having intensely-felt regrets (Landman, 1987; Wrosch, Bauer, & Scheier, 2005).

In addition, when people review their past, they may ruminate about their "possible self" – the person that they might have become "if only" they did or did not do what they have come to regret. Further, when people do have major regrets, they often use these regrets as key elements of a "life narrative" or explanation of how they have arrived at their current place in life. And when people use the idea of "what might have been" as a standard, they place their well-being at risk. They are likely to over-idealize the possible and imagine what might have been as more satisfying than whatever has actually occurred. As a result, they are likely to feel frustrated, disappointed, sad, guilty, and remorseful (Markus & Nurius, 1986; Landman, 1987).

Life-regrets defined

Life-regrets can be defined both etymologically and based on the psychological literature. Etymologically, the word "regret" is present in old French and is similar to the English word "bewail". It is also present in Scandinavian and similar to the old Norse word "grata", which means "to weep". Thus, what seems to be the essential commonality among these word roots is loss – when people experience a regret, they seem to be mourning for something that they wished for, that they imagine would have occurred if they had acted differently than they did. What is also suggested is that a regret tends to trigger a need to lament – to feel sorry for oneself and experience guilt, disappointment, or pain, either over what the person chose not to do (i.e. an act of omission), or chose to do (i.e. an act of commission) (Landman, 1987; Trumble, 2002).

Psychologically, a regret is said to occur when a person makes a comparison between two possibilities, one that has actually occurred and one that did not, and following the comparison, imagines that the choice they did not make is better and preferable to the choice they did make (McQueen, 2017). As a result, the person typically feels angry, helpless, and sad, and ruminates about the alternative not chosen, usually thinking such thoughts as "if only I" or "I might have" (Landman, 1987).

Well-being is affected differently by regrets of commission compared to regrets of omission. People tend to be more upset initially by regrets about what they did than by regrets about what they did not do. As time passes, however, especially in old age, people's upset over what they did not do is likely to become relatively more powerful and play a stronger role in the life narrative the person constructs. Thus, people are more likely to be dissatisfied and distressed by thoughts of what might have been as they imagine the "road not taken" (Gilovich & Medvec, 1995).

A person is especially likely to be distressed if they subsequently acquire evidence that they would have been successful in achieving or avoiding the desired outcome that they wish had occurred. And, relative to regrets over actions that they did take, regrets over what a person did not do are open-ended; they are limited only by the strength of a person's imagination. As a result, again especially in old age, it is relatively easy for a person to be disappointed when they compare their actual life to this imagined, often idealized outcome that they now wish they had acted to attain (Gilovich & Medvec, 1995).

The impact of life-regrets on well-being

As would be expected, a person's subjective well-being is likely to be relatively lower if they ruminate about past choices that they made – on the things that they had hoped to accomplish or experience in their life and especially, what they feel would now be better "if" they only had made the alternative choice. Thus, when people do not resolve their regrets- when they remain preoccupied with what might have been, they are likely to have a relatively lower level of life satisfaction and a relatively higher level of negative emotions (Bauer, Wrosch, & Jobin, 2008).

As has been noted, age also seems to play a role. The older people are, the more likely it is that they will be preoccupied with intense regrets because they are more likely to be aware of the limited time that they now have available to achieve the alternative goals that they wished for; realize they have fewer opportunities to undo the consequences of what they have come to regret; and believe they have fewer personal resources to affect their regrets. As a consequence, at older ages, when people dwell on their regrets they are more likely to feel helpless and depressed and have less motivation to maintain their health, particularly if they are unable to identify alternative goals to work towards (Wrosch, Bauer, & Scheier, 2005).

The following vignette illustrates several of the key ideas noted in the selective review of the literature:

That did not go as expected. He thought he was being the good planner. Six months before his planned retirement, he would see his physician, get a health exam, and then with his expected "clean bill of health", fill in the next, much anticipated chapter of his post-work life. Instead, James, age 64, has just been told that his PSA test was abnormally high, and along with the findings on his physical exam, that it was likely he had prostate cancer. The urologist he saw the next day confirmed that this was the case and said that the progression of the disease could be slowed but not stopped. When James asked the physician what "slowed" meant, the physician was unclear and said they were talking about years not months.

Numb, James felt that life had just played a joke on him. He had worked 70 to 80 hours a week in his father's business since he was 20, a business that he eventually took over, and while now wealthy, he had never taken the time to have a regular life – to spend evenings home with his family, to go on family vacations, and to participate in the important and unimportant events that made up his two daughters' lives.

He had intended for all this to change – once he retired he would no longer have to criticize himself for being a crummy dad and husband – no longer be the admired stranger to his daughters and now his granddaughters, the one whose only role was to provide money whenever anyone wanted something; and no longer have to be the missing partner whose absence caused his wife Jill to act as if she were a single mother and grandmother.

Angry, James imagined how life with his family might have been if he had retired at 50 like his friend Ted. He couldn't really explain why he hadn't. He had enough money. Maybe he was just programmed like his father to work. Over and over he kept wondering if there was enough time left to make things different.

Part two: Ways of maintaining well-being in the face of life-regrets

The following ideas and strategies can be used by clinicians if a person raises one or more of the following concerns during a clinical encounter.

Helping the person examine and articulate what they regret

When responding to questions about a person's history, the person may describe having strong regrets, regrets that they feel with age they are less and less likely to be able to rectify. A clinician can offer to help the person examine their regrets and better understand the factors that influenced the choices that were made (Wrosch & Heckhausen, 2002). The clinician can point out that, while it may no longer be possible to change the conditions that led to the choice – to make external changes – a person is likely to be less distressed about regrets and have a higher level of well-being if they can make internal changes – change the way they think about what they regret, and especially reconsider and reassess the actual degree of personal control and responsibility that they had at the time they were faced with the choice.

Thus the clinician can explain that, in contrast to what Lady Macbeth famously said, "Things without remedy should be without regard; what is done is done" (quoted in Landman, 1987, p. 154), it is often beneficial for a person to think about what they regret. While there is also some support for Lady Macbeth's view, the clinician can point out that, excessively focusing and ruminating about a past choice is especially maladaptive and, overall, people are still more likely to have a higher level of well-being if they can be self-aware and learn from, rather than try to not think about, the choices that they have made or did not make (Butler, 1963; Torges, Stewart, & Nolen-Hoeksema, 2008).

The clinician can further explain that when people take the time to reflect on their actions, they are found to be more satisfied with their life; better able to understand their life story and the factors that influenced their actions; better able to reappraise what had occurred and forgive themselves; and, perhaps most importantly, more likely to identify goals that matter to them and that they can still work to achieve in the present (Torges et al., 2008).

The clinician can explain that people might try to cope differently with regrets of omission and regrets of commission. A person is likely to be less distressed in regard to regrets of omission (i.e. the choices they did not make made but wished they had), if they consider what they can still do to directly or indirectly fulfill the objective they were seeking by making this choice. With regard to reflecting on regrets of commission (i.e. the choices a person made but wishes they had not), the clinician can note that a person's well-being is likely to be higher if they can find ways to challenge the degree to which they feel they are blameworthy (Gilovich & Medvec, 1995).

The clinician can also suggest that the person consider writing about their regrets. When they search for words to describe the nature and circumstances of their regrets, they are likely to be more self-aware and have greater clarity about what they are specifically regretting. They may also be better able to posit an alternative, more forgiving explanation for what they did or did not do (Pennebaker, 1997). In addition, the clinician can explain that the act of writing – of explicitly expressing what they need to "lament about"– may allow the person to acknowledge and let out, rather than avoid and inhibit, what has upset them. As a result, the pent up emotions that the person has been storing might be released and their distress reduced (Wrosch, Bauer, Miller, & Lupien, 2007).

Helping the person examine if they were blameworthy

If a person is highly self-critical of a past choice, a clinician can offer to help the person decide if they are in fact blameworthy. The clinician can point out that when people experience and ruminate about what they regret, especially what they can no longer affect, they often attempt to explain or justify what they did or did not do. They are especially likely to attribute what they have come to regret to a personal limitation, to events outside their control, or to both.

The clinician can note that the specific reason the person attaches to their choice will differentially affect their emotional reactions. For example, when people feel they were too cowardly to do something they now wish that they had, they are likely to feel ashamed and remorseful; while when people feel that circumstances, or external events, are the cause of their regret (e.g. their family was too poor to afford to send them to school), they are likely to feel disappointed and sad (Bauer & Wrosch, 2011).

To help a person counter their self-criticisms, the clinician can describe the Justified Decision Perspective (McQueen, 2017). Using this perspective, the clinician explains, the person tries to makes sure that a person is judging themselves in regard to a decision that they have made using only the circumstance and reasons that existed at the time they made the decision, and also not judging themselves using reasons or circumstances that arose after the decision was made.

If a person does conclude that he or she is blameworthy, to help lessen their self-blame and increase their sense of well-being, the clinician can point out the value of being self-compassionate – of exerting effort to understand and if possible sympathize with the reasons they had for making their choice and the importance of extending to themselves the nonjudgmental kindness and concern that they might extend to a close friend who was in a similar circumstance. Thus, if they were trying to be kind to a friend, the clinician can explain, they might encourage the friend to forgive him or herself and recognize that they are simply human, that is, imperfect and fallible (Neff, 2003).

The use of silver lining, downward social comparison, and realism

To help a person focus away from what they feel they have lost by what either they did or did not do, the clinician can suggest they consider applying the notion of "silver linings" to combat their regrets – to identify the positives that may have resulted from the choices that they made, ways that they have actually profited from what they did or did not do. For example, with the clinician's help, the person may be able to appreciate all the things that they have learned from their regrettable choice, or all the things they have accomplished by not doing "X" and instead by doing "Y" (Gilovich & Medvec, 1995).

When a person looks for silver linings, the clinician can emphasize, the person is likely to feel a rise in well-being because they are now focusing on what they feel grateful for rather than focusing on what they feel is missing. To amplify the positive still more, the clinician can mention the strategy of making a "downward social comparison". The person might compare their life with someone similar to themselves and note how much better off their life turned out than the other person's, even though they made the choice they now regret (Bauer, Wrosch, & Jobin, 2008).

Finally, the clinician can suggest still another that way the person may combat negative thoughts about what they regret. They can make sure that they are not over-idealizing what "might have been"; that is, that they are not focusing exclusively on the benefits that they imagine would have followed "if only" they had done or not done what they now regret. Instead, they can try to exert effort to be realistic rather than wishful in predicting what might have been, and remember the actual circumstances or obstacles that were present at the time.

Providing a key take-away message: To seize the day

The clinician can emphasize that perhaps the most essential strategy, not only for managing regrets but, as mentioned, for coping with many of the challenges attached to aging, is to be accepting, to recognize what they can and cannot change. Thus, as the famous psychologist Erik Erikson said, people need to acknowledge and accept their past choices if they are to avoid despair and experience a sense of integrity, especially in the final stages of their life (Erikson, Erikson, & Kivnik, 1986). By doing so, Erikson went on to say, a person may not only be less upset over what they have done or not done but also may be able to create a new focus; they are more likely to try to "seize the day" and create alternative goals that allow them to live in the present and fulfill what they now desire while they still have the time to do so.

The following vignette illustrates several of the strategies that have been mentioned:

James decided to consult a psychologist. During the appointment he described how his life was now in turmoil, in part because of the cancer diagnosis he had just received, and in part because of his poor planning. He told the psychologist that he had sacrificed family time and fun for a future pay-off that he now thought he would have much less time to enjoy. After James detailed what had occurred, the psychologist said he was impressed by James' understanding of why he did what he did; that his reasons did not seem self-serving but loving and at great personal cost. The psychologist went on to say that while James seemed exceptionally good at being self-aware, he seemed exceptionally bad at showing self-compassion. He also seemed to be making a thinking error. He was failing to recognize that at the time that he made the choices that he now regrets, he looked at the future differently than he does now after being given the cancer diagnosis. The psychologist concluded by saying that he thought James could still be the parent that he wanted to be and might start by meeting with his daughters and telling them what he was now thinking and feeling.

After reflecting on what he and the psychologist discussed, James made several decisions. He told his work associates about his health and that he was going to retire. He scheduled the first of 12 radiation treatments that he had been prescribed to slow his illness, and he asked his daughters to join him for lunch.

Once seated at the table with his daughters, James explained that partly because of his illness and partly because he had been reviewing his life in anticipation of retirement, he felt that he owed them an apology. He had prioritized making money instead of spending time with them. While he told them he did it to make sure they were okay, he said he had failed to be the dad he now wishes that he had been – a dad who was an everyday part of their life, who attended parent-teacher nights, who drove them to their friends' houses, and who knew the things that were most important to them.

James told his daughters that he realized he had worked so hard out of a fear; that unless he did, he worried his business would fail and then he wouldn't be able to make sure that they and their mother were safe. His daughters, Stacy and Susan, listened, and in almost identical words, told him that they did feel bad that he had missed so many important events, yet they both said that they knew that he loved them and had done what he did for them. They told him that going forward, they wanted to see him frequently and that what was especially important was that their children could get to know their grandpa.

Reflecting on the meeting afterwards, James felt lucky. His partner, who had worked the same long hours that he had, died suddenly last year. He never had the chance to make up for what he too may have regretted. James also thought that while he was not the father that he should have been, in many ways he could be proud of the opportunities and sense of comfort that his hard work had produced for his family. He then tried to imagine the kind of father and grandfather he now would aspire to be. Almost immediately he thought that he would like to imitate his father's father – like his grandfather, he would be interested in what his daughters and grandchildren had to say and take delight in their accomplishments.

Summary

It is likely as people age that they will periodically look back, review their major life choices and actions, and experience a sense of regret for some of the things that they either did or did not do. As a result, their sense of well-being can be threatened; they may ruminate about this alternative choice, imagine how their life might have been significantly better if they had chosen it, and as a result, be self-critical and distressed.

When people express regrets and feel that they can no longer make external changes to affect a past situation to the degree that they wish, a clinician can suggest that the person focus on making internal changes. Towards this end, the clinician can encourage the person to try to be as objective as possible and see if they can alter their perceptions and attitudes about what has occurred; note any "silver linings" or benefits that have resulted from their regretted choice; focus on what they can still feel grateful for; recognize how, in important ways, they may be still better off than others they know, even though they have made the choice that they now regret; and finally, not over-idealize what they imagine the alternative outcome might have been.

If people continue to feel blameworthy, the clinician can also suggest that they try to challenge the validity of their self-criticisms – to make sure that they are judging themselves based on what occurred at the time of their choice and not on what has occurred subsequently. By having made this thoughtful examination, the clinician can explain the person is more likely to better understand their motives and the context that was present at the time of their choice, and as a result, will be more likely to be self-compassionate and self-forgiving.

Finally, the clinician can highlight the need to be self-reflective in order to learn as much as possible from the experience of feeling regretful, and most importantly, use this information to "seize the day" and work to achieve goals in the present.

Chapter 6

Still another challenge

Age-associated memory loss

Part one: A selective review of the literature

Overview

People as they age are likely to experience some degree of age-associated memory loss which will challenge their ability to maintain a sense of well-being. When a person is unable to remember as well as they did in the past they are at risk of feeling embarrassed, self-critical, less in control, disinterested in socializing, and less motivated to learn. In addition, they may become frightened that their memory problems will worsen and are a prelude to what is usually experienced as terrifying – the possibility of developing dementia (Parikh, Troyer, Malone, & Murphy, 2015; Verhaeghen, Geraerts, & Marcoen, 2000).

Memory and aging

When older people are surveyed, memory loss is one of the most feared and frequently mentioned complaints (Dixon, Rust, Feltmate, & See, 2007). People are likely to be highly aware of occasions in which they forget such things as where they put their keys; the date of an appointment that they had scheduled; why they walked into a room; what they just read or heard; a word that they were about to say; or the name of an acquaintance (Parikh et al., 2015; Park, O'Connell, & Thompson, 2003).

About 40% of people aged 65 or older are likely to have specific memory impairments and, occasionally, forget specific events and experiences in their recent past as well as specific upcoming events and experiences (Koivisto et al., 1995). In addition, as they get older they are also likely to experience a decline in the speed with which they process information; they are aware that they need more time to think about the meaning of the information that they have been exposed to and more time to recall the information. They are also likely to experience a decline in their ability to simultaneously store and manipulate information and as a result, tend to substitute one memory with a similar one (e.g. calling a son by a grandson's name), become distracted, and when they try to retrieve and express information, have it become stuck on the "tip of their tongue" (Koivisto et al., 1995).

Yet even though with age most people are occasionally more forgetful and process information more slowly, they usually still can recall and describe incidents that they experience; independently and successfully carry out everyday activities; maintain their usual level of judgment and decision-making; find their way to a desired location even if they do get momentarily disoriented; and successfully maintain a conversation even if they periodically have difficulty finding a particular word to express what they had intended to say (Park et al., 2003; D'Esposito & Gazzaley, 2011).

Episodic versus semantic memory changes

To explain this variability in the type and degree of various memory deficits affected by age, researchers often use a memory systems perspective, a theory that proposes that there are multiple systems of memory that "age" at different rates (Dixon et al., 2007). The two memory systems said to be most relevant when explaining the effects of aging have been labeled episodic and semantic memory (Hicks, Alexander, & Bahr, 2018). Episodic memory refers to a person's memory for personally experienced events or information, such as when a person is introduced to someone and tries to remember the name of the person they were introduced to, where they placed an object, what they heard in a conversation the day before, or when in a store without a list, what they intended to purchase. There is an abundance of evidence that indicates that episodic memory declines as people get older (Dixon et al., 2007; Hicks et al., 2018). For normal aging adults, the magnitude of these age-associated changes is relatively gradual until the mid-seventies, after which there is a relatively rapid decline (Dixon et al., 2004).

Semantic memory refers to a person's memory for acquiring and retaining generic facts, knowledge, and beliefs (e.g. knowing that football is a sport, how to use scissors, the color of an object, or the capital of a country). Unlike the decline in episodic memory, perhaps because of an older person's accumulated experience and knowledge, older adults are able to remember this type of information as well as younger adults, although as stated earlier, they may need more time to access and process the information (Backman & Nilsson, 1996).

Age-associated memory loss and well-being

A person's distress over memory loss tends to be based less on objective indications of the nature and frequency of their memory problems and more on their perceptions – the extent to which they believe that their memory is markedly poorer than it was in the past and markedly poorer than the memory of their peers (Verhaeghen et al., 2000; Frank et al., 2006; Parikh, Troyer,

Malone, & Murphy, 2015). As mentioned, people often become frightened if they perceive that their memory problems are worsening and often worry that their memory problems might increase and become like the memory problems of someone with Alzheimer's disease, a person who is dependent and unaware of both who they are and who others are that have mattered to them (Frank et al., 2006).

When an older person believes that they are likely to have trouble remembering, they are less likely to place themselves in situations in which there are high memory demands and when in these situations and do have memory lapses, frequently experience frustration, embarrassment, and shame. As a consequence, older people who believe that they are likely to fail to remember someone's name might avoid being in social situations where they expect to be introduced and then have to socialize with people whose names they may have forgotten (Dixon et al., 2007). Thus they are at risk of becoming withdrawn and receiving less social support than they have in the past at a time when such support would be especially helpful (Frank et al., 2006; Joosten-Weyn, Kessels, Rikert, Geleijns-Lanting, & Kraaimaat., 2008; Parikh et al., 2015).

This increased risk of avoidance can also interfere with an older person's sense of well-being because they may seek fewer opportunities to learn and experience personal growth (Miller & Lachman, 1999; Verhaeghen et al., 2000), or when in a learning situation, may exert less effort and give up quickly when they feel intellectually challenged (Dixon et al., 2007).

The following vignette illustrates several of the key ideas noted in the selective review of the literature:

The movie ended and Charlotte sat, deep in thought. She agreed with the friend who had recommended the movie, that the acting was great. Yet for her, it was almost unbearable to watch- to see the main character gradually developing signs of early onset dementia- first, forgetting a word, then losing her way even though she was in a place that she had been many times before, and eventually, being unable to recognize her own daughter.

"Would this be her?" Since she turned 69 last May, she noticed that she was having difficulty at times finding the right word, last week spent about an hour looking for her car in the mall garage, and this morning, when she went to get the paper, felt embarrassed when her neighbor greeted her and for a minute she couldn't remember the neighbor's name. Probably what was most upsetting was what happened during the book group. After she had asked a question, Jane leaned towards her and whispered, "you are repeating yourself; you asked the same question a little while ago". Thinking about that moment was excruciating and she wasn't sure if she would attend the next meeting of the group.

Hearing about what happened to her second cousin, Mary, had added to her worry. Her cousin had been diagnosed with dementia when she was 70, only about 6 months older than Charlotte is now. Mary had been having more and more difficulty taking care of herself and after wandering off several times, was placed in a long-term care facility.

Part two: Strategies to manage concerns about memory loss

The following ideas and strategies can be used by clinicians if a person raises concerns about their memory during a clinical encounter.

Providing reality information

When a person expresses upset about memory failure, a clinician can provide a realistic understanding of the typical changes in memory that occur with age – that most people inevitably and gradually decline in their memory for personally relevant facts and events, such as where they placed something or what they were intending to do next and display relatively little to no change in their ability to retain generic facts, knowledge, and personal beliefs (Dixon et al., 2004; Dixon et al., 2007). A clinician needs to also highlight that these statements are generalities and that there is a great deal of variation among specific individuals so that many older people are able to retain their cognitive capacities by finding ways to compensate for their memory difficulties (Dixon et al., 2007).

Suggesting a fact-based self-assessment

If a person describes a number of incidents in which they have felt embarrassed or especially frustrated by their memory difficulties and seems significantly distressed about what these difficulties connote (e.g. they think they may be developing dementia), the clinician can explain that it is important to gather facts rather than rely on perceptions. Towards this end, the clinician can suggest that the person keep track of the actual nature of their memory lapses and, for example, each evening, for a period of about two weeks, write down the type and degree of the memory lapses that have occurred, and the amount of interference that these memory lapses have caused in their ability to independently carry out daily tasks.

The clinician can explain, that with the clinician's help, after this data is acquired the person could use the data to compare the memory lapses that they have noted to typical examples of normal memory lapses (i.e. occasionally forgetting where things were left, names of acquaintances, an appointment, why they entered a room, and what they were about to say); evaluate the degree to which these memory lapses interfere with their ability to perform everyday tasks; and, if the data continues to be collected over a period of time, determine if their memory is significantly declining.

Helping to decide when a consultation is needed

After reviewing the data, the clinician may be able to reassure the person that their memory lapses do not seem to signify a clinical problem – they are similar to the type of memory lapses that most people their age experience, do not seem significantly different in nature or frequency to the memory lapses the person described experiencing over the last few years, and do not interfere with their ability to carry out daily tasks.

If the data is either ambiguous or indicates that there may be a clinical problem, or if the person remains highly concerned even though the data does not suggest a clinical problem, the clinician can suggest the person go for a consultation with someone who has expertise in the diagnosis of memory problems. The clinician can explain that during the appointment the consultant will conduct a formal assessment to determine if a memory problem is present, and if so, will attempt to clarify the nature of the problem and propose a course of action.

The clinician can explain that it would be helpful, if the person has collected facts about their memory lapses, that they bring them to the consultation and, given their doubts about their memory, that they ask someone who knows them well to accompany them to the visit to provide background information and to listen along with them to what they are told.

In addition to telling the consultant about the frequency and type of memory lapses that they have been experiencing, the clinician can suggest that the person be prepared to tell how the memory problems are manifested; the degree and type of interference the memory problems cause in carrying out everyday tasks; when the memory concerns began, any changes that have occurred, and if changes have occurred, whether they have been gradual or sudden; the names and dates of anyone who has been consulted about the memory problems in the past and what was said during these consultations; any medications that they are taking or which have been taken; the amount and type of alcohol and drugs they are using or which have been used; any injuries that have occurred, especially head injuries; any emotional crises that have occurred, such as the loss of a spouse or child; and lastly, if they have been experiencing a high degree of sadness or anxiety.

Preparing for lapses in memory

If a person describes feeling self-critical and embarrassed when they have memory concerns, for example, when they lose track of what they intend to say, cannot find their keys as they are leaving a friend's house, or have no recollection of where they parked their car as they are walking towards the parking lot with someone, the clinician can reassure the person that these feelings are fairly common. The clinician can then point out that people are less likely to be distressed and better able to manage their negative emotions at these times, if they practice using "implementation intentions" (Gollwitzer, 1999) – sets of self-instructions that they can develop, rehearse in advance, and employ in situations in which they predict they will be stressed or upset. In a sense they are pre-plans and sets of goals that allow the person to delineate in detail how they ideally wish to behave at challenging times (Brier, 2015).

If the person is interested in employing this technique, the clinician could then coach the person in its use. The clinician explains that the person employs a conditional, if-then phrase, "**If** situation X arises, **then** I will do Y", and illustrates its use as follows: A person is anticipating that they will be unable to remember a desired word. They decide to practice saying to themselves, "**If** I can't think of the word I want to say, **then** I will take a deep breath. I will say give me a minute and try to think of a synonym. If I am still stuck, I will say, it's not that important and then I will switch the topic.". The clinician can tell the person that it is often helpful to review the plan periodically before trying it out. In addition, while doing so, they can visualize as vividly and in as much detail as possible, past occasions where they have felt embarrassed or at a loss, and then contrast that image with the image of their feeling better having a plan that will help them not feel at a loss.

The clinician might also mention that when people are self-conscious about memory lapses, they may be tempted to avoid situations in which they anticipate feeling ashamed or embarrassed and suggest that employing an implementation intention might again be helpful. The person might say to themselves, for example, "If 'X' makes a face when I forget a word, then I will say to myself, calm down, you can deal with this, and either try to find an alternative word or change the topic." The clinician can stress that it is very important that the person face rather than avoid their discomfort because if they do withdraw and avoid situations when they anticipate embarrassment, they are likely to become more isolated. They will then risk having less support at a time when they especially need it.

Helping the person learn memory compensation strategies

The clinician can also offer to help the person learn a variety of memory compensation strategies to help minimize the effects of memory loss and to gain evidence that they are still able to influence and lessen their memory problems. The clinician can explain that there is a great deal of research to show that the use of memory compensation strategies is likely to reduce both the frequency of forgetting and the impact of forgetting on managing daily tasks (Simon, Yokomizo, & Bottino, 2012; Willis & Belleville, 2016; Gollwitzer, 1999; Troyer, Murphy, Anderson, Moscovitch, & Craik, 2008; Simon et al., 2012).

The clinician could then review the most frequently recommended strategies, starting with the importance of being as mentally active as possible. The clinician can share that most experts support the idea that engaging in mentally stimulating activities as a person gets older is helpful and believe that intellectual engagement may prevent or at least alter the rate of mental decline associated with aging. The clinician can then provide examples of typical mental activities that people generally choose such as: playing challenging games like bridge and chess, completing crossword puzzles, assembling puzzles, learning a foreign language or how to play a musical instrument, and taking a class in an area of interest (Salthouse, 2006; Simon et al., 2012).

The clinician can then present another highly recommended memory compensatory strategy – setting up and keeping to routines and placing things in set locations. When people carry out actions in the same order, at the same time, and in the same way, the clinician can explain, they eventually do these actions automatically or habitually and as a result, they are more likely to remember to do what they intended to do. People are more likely to remember to take their medication, for example, if they attempt to do so at the same time each day, in a set order. The clinician can repeat that when creating routines it is helpful to carry them out in a structured and predictable setting – to make sure that the environment is uncluttered and organized, and that things are placed in and returned to the same spot. For example they might put their keys on a particular hook in a particular part of a specific room and put each of their glasses in a specific glasses case that they keep in a specific location.

If the person displays an interest in a more detailed explanation as to why routines help, the clinician can spell out that when a person uses a routine, they strengthen memory associations. They establish and increase the availability of such cues as the time of day, what comes earlier in a sequence, and contextual cues. As a result, the number of elements that support their memory is increased, and by regularly engaging in the routine, the person strengthens the connection between the elements of what they want to remember. Further, when people keep to a routine, they do not have to make choices. As a consequence, they reduce the mental effort they are exerting and thereby the demand made on memory storage (Wood & Runger, 2016).

Teaching about the use of external memory aids

The clinician lastly might describe what is perhaps the most frequently recommended strategy to shore up a person's memory as they get older – external memory aids or tools that provide "reminders" as to what needs to be remembered. The clinician can explain that using a memory aid is probably the most efficient way a person can increase their ability to remember planned actions and intentions (Wang & Perez-Quinones, 2014), and point out that it is not uncommon for older adults to have developed their own ways of compensating for memory loss. Therefore, before the clinician makes suggestions, he or she might inquire if the person has developed some ways on their own to cope with memory lapses in the past and if they have, ask them to describe how successful what they have tried has been.

The clinician can mention that the most common external aids include the use of smart phone apps, to-do lists, daily planners, calendars, an always available notepad and pen, a list of frequently needed information, and alarms that signal when there is either a need to remember something or do something (e.g. keep an appointment or take a medicine). Still another external reminder the clinician can mention is the enlistment of someone's help in reminding them of upcoming important dates and tasks (Dixon et al., 2007).

A final cluster of tools: Personal association, acronyms, and attention management

The clinician can also review three more strategies that people find helpful to compensate for memory loss. The first involves the use of personal associations. To help a person increase their recall, the clinician explains, a person might think of something that rhymes with what they wish to remember, or picture something that they feel captures its essence. If a person wanted to remember where they had placed an apple, for example, they might picture how round and very red it is and its placement on the corner of the kitchen table and if a person wants to remember that their flight departs at 2 pm, they might picture an airplane and focus on its two wings.

The clinician can also describe the use of acronyms – to use the first letters of each word in a phrase to remember it. For example, to remember the phrase, thank god it is Friday, a person might create the acronym TGIF. A final strategy the clinician can mention is attention management – ways a person can selectively and strategically focus on what they want to remember and, with effort, allocate as much of their attention as they can towards a specific "target". For example, if a person wants to remember where they parked their car, they might pause, concentrate solely on where their car is located, and as described earlier, make a link or association to a sign that is nearby. As they do, they might also concentrate and repeat what they wish to remember at increasingly spaced intervals, especially if it is new information such as a phone number or a set of directions.

The following vignette illustrates several of the strategies that have been mentioned:

Charlotte was both looking forward to and dreading her annual health exam. She hoped she would get reassurance about her memory problems yet knew that she would feel upset when the doctor pointed out all the ways that her body had deteriorated since last year's visit. Charlotte had kept track of the times she forgot things and intended to ask the doctor if he thought what was going on was normal or abnormal.

Once seated at the appointment and asked about any health concerns she was having, Charlotte told the doctor about the forgetting and handed him the paper on which she had written dates when she had memory lapses and the details of what occurred. Charlotte also mentioned what had happened to her cousin and asked whether, because of having a cousin who developed dementia, she was more at risk of developing dementia. As the doctor reviewed the list with her, he asked how she handled each of the situations that she had noted and if she was still able to successfully do what she needed to do on each of these occasions.

At the end of the visit, the doctor told Charlotte he felt that both the type and amount of her memory lapses were normal for someone her age, and that having a second cousin who developed dementia did not increase her risk for the disorder. To her surprise and relief, he also told her that nothing much had changed since last year's visit and handed her a brochure. It was developed by the National Institute of Mental Health, he said, and it described ways of coping with memory lapses as people age. He added that many of his patients found it helpful.

In the weeks following the doctor's appointment, while Charlotte felt less worried about her memory, occasionally she would still get anxious; for example, one time when she heard about a neighbor showing signs of dementia and another time, when watching a movie in which a character was portrayed as having a severe memory problem. Charlotte decided to try out some of the ideas mentioned in the brochure. One idea had to do with coping with embarrassment. When you forget something, it said in the brochure, try not to beat yourself up; instead it advised to be compassionate and understanding – for example, it suggested saying "it stinks to get old but I have to accept that this is the way it is".

Also mentioned in the brochure was the idea of giving feedback to people who thought they were being helpful when you had a memory lapse but instead upset you. With the book group scheduled for next week, Charlotte decided that she would try out this suggestion and say something to Jane. She wanted to say it in a way that didn't make it seem like such a big deal and make things very uncomfortable afterwards. She came up with the idea that, before the group, she would tell Jane that she wanted to talk. She would then first tell her that she knew Jane had been trying to be helpful at the last group when she told her that she was repeating herself. She would say that she thought that Jane made the comment so that Charlotte wouldn't again put herself in a position where she might be embarrassed. Charlotte would then go on to say that what Jane said actually had the opposite effect; it made her feel more self-conscious. Charlotte would end the conversation by saying that she was now aware of her memory problems and didn't need them pointed out.

Several other ideas mentioned in the brochure also seemed worth trying. One had to do with always putting things in the same place, especially things you regularly wound up searching for, like her phone, keys, and watch. As suggested, Charlotte bought small, pretty dishes, one for each possession she wanted to keep track of. Each night she would place the object in its "designated" dish. Also, as suggested, she started to use reminders. She began to enter into her smartphone all the things that she needed to do as well as her appointments; then, both at the start of each day and before each meal, she would check her to-do list and calendar.

Gradually, Charlotte noticed that in fact she was forgetting less. She felt proud of the way that she had handled things and felt reassured. If something was really wrong with her memory, doing a few simple things would not have made such a big difference.

Summary

With increasing age, most people experience an age-related decline in episodic memory – memory for personally experienced events or information but not semantic memory – memory for generic facts, knowledge, and beliefs. When people do experience memory failure, it threatens their sense of well-being by challenging their self-esteem, desire to engage in social interactions, ability to experience personal growth, and sense of personal control.

A clinician can explain that a person's perception of changes in their memory has a relatively greater effect on their well-being than any objective changes that may be occurring. The clinician can also point out that when people perceive changes in memory, they are likely to become anxious and worry that they will develop Alzheimer's disease. At times, they can also feel self-conscious, anticipate that they might have a memory lapse when around others, and be tempted to avoid social situations in which the memory lapse occurred. The clinician can explain that there is a danger attached to giving in to this understandable temptation; by doing so they risk reducing the availability of social support at a time when they are especially likely to need it.

The clinician can also describe another risk: When a person loses confidence in their ability to remember, they may feel less motivated to pursue learning opportunities, and if they do cease to engage in such experiences, they are less likely to experience personal growth and more likely to experience a decline in their level of well-being.

The clinician can present a range of strategies that a person can employ to clarify the nature of their memory problem and to compensate and lessen the negative effects of their memory difficulties. Thus, the clinician can teach such strategies as pre-planning for occasions when memory lapses occur; engaging in activities to "exercise" memory; establishing and maintaining routines; using external memory aids; employing personal associations; and regulating attention.

Chapter 7

Aging, well-being, and old-old age

Part one: A selective review of the literature

Young-old and old-old age defined

There has been a striking increase in the number of people who reach late life and have to adapt to the physical, emotional, and social changes that exist at this time (Menninger, 1999). Because what is considered old age now covers a much greater age span, it is important to distinguish the needs, pressures, and circumstances that people face early in old age from the needs, pressures, and circumstances that people face late in old age (Martin, Kliegel, Rott, Poon, and Johnson, 2008).

Using the labels young-old and old-old age proposed by the World Health Organization (WHO, 1963), people between the ages of 60 and 74 are considered young-old or elderly, while people who are 75 and older are considered old-old or aged. Thus, WHO uses chronological age as the central criterion to make this distinction, consistent with the obvious finding that the older a person is, the more their cellular, organ, and biological systems decline and the more they will be (and feel) old-old.

And consistent with WHO's proposed distinction, 68% of people aged 16 to 64 report that they are in good health compared to 40% of people aged 65 and older. Also consistent with the WHO distinction is the finding that rates of chronic illness increase significantly after age 60 (Tinker, 1993). While reasonable to use as a marker, however, chronological age is a highly imprecise dividing line between young-old and old-old age, given the tremendous differences that exist in rates of aging among people of the same age. As a result, to make a meaningful and reliable distinction between young-old and old-old age people need to use two additional criteria.

The first criterion is a person's biological/physical health age – their "reserve capacity" or ability to be resilient, "bounce back", and function adequately in the face of deficits, disabilities, and losses (Karasik, Demissie, Cupples, & Kiel, 2005). Using this criterion, the start of old age is considered to be the time when a person's biological capacity has decreased to the point where they can no longer either maintain or restore their biological and adaptive "homeostasis". As a consequence, the person is more likely to have an increasing amount of difficulty independently managing everyday tasks and is less likely to experience significant gains in the quality of their life (Mendoza-Nunez, 2016). Instead, going forward, they almost exclusively are likely to experience decrements and the balance between gains and losses therefore is likely to be tilted dramatically towards losses.

The second criterion to indicate the start of old-old age is a person's subjective or perceived age – how young or old the person feels relative to their chronological age. People tend to form a judgment of their subjective age based on both the social and cultural cues that they receive and the biomedical "messages" that they detect from their bodily systems. With regard to feedback they receive from others, people are more likely to see themselves as old-old when they continuously and predominantly receive messages that support the idea that they are old-old, especially if they experience these messages as hurtful and are already sensitive to this type of feedback (i.e. they already are upset and self-conscious about their lack of energy, wrinkles, or sagging skin) (Levy, 2009; Stephan, Sutin, & Terracciano, 2015).

With regard to biomedical messages, people are more likely to feel old-old when they continuously experience pain, fatigue, breathlessness, a lack of muscle strength, or difficulty with their memory; and are especially likely to feel that they have entered old-old-age when these two sources of data align – when others respond to them as if they are old and when they are highly and continuously aware of the increased number of deficits and disabilities that they have (Mendoza-Nunez, 2016).

Key psychological distinctions between young-old and old-old age

In young-old age, while people are likely to experience some degree of decline and deterioration, they tend to still feel that they are more or less the same person that they have always been (Gana, Alaphillipe, & Bailly, 2004). Further, if people adjust what they do and how they do it, in young-old age they often are still able to compensate for the physical and mental limitations that they are experiencing. As a result, they are able to continue to enjoy many of the activities that they have enjoyed in the past (Baltes & Baltes, 1990). Lastly, in young-old age people are likely to still feel relatively independent and efficacious and are viewed in this way by most others (Weiss, Sassenberg, & Freund, 2013).

In old-old age, in contrast, people tend to not feel that they are the same person that they used to be. Their awareness of their physical decline, along with their accumulating health problems, are likely to make them feel less able to overcome or rebound from obstacles and setbacks, manage everyday tasks, and successfully carry out many of the activities that they have previously valued (Staudinger, Marsiske, & Baltes, 1995). Finally, in old-old age, people are more likely to feel dependent and identify with the negative stereotypes that are typically attached to the elderly (e.g. dependent, impaired, and frail) (Levy, 2009).

Old-old age and well-being

During old-old age people are likely to focus on the limited time that they have remaining to live (Lang and Carstensen, 2002; Palgi & Shmotkin, 2010) and as a result are likely to experience a change in their temporal perspective. Instead of considering the future, they are more likely to focus on the present-on what is realistically achievable in the near-term. They are also more likely to focus on the payoffs that they feel are emotionally meaningful to them, such as creating a legacy and experiencing closeness with others, particularly with others who they view as special to them and who they want to be most remembered by (Carstensen, Isaacowitz, & Charles, 1999; Lennings, 2000).

In addition to a preoccupation with mortality, another challenge to a person's sense of well-being in old-old age is the increasing number of functional limitations and chronic diseases that are likely to be present which can interfere with mobility, the ability to carry out self-care skills, and their sense of personal control. Because people are less able to rely on ourselves to carry out everyday tasks or manage any functional disabilities that they may have (Rodriquez-Diaz, Perez-Marfil, & Cruz-Quintana, 2016), they are likely to have difficulty maintaining a positive identity. As a result, in old-old age people often view themselves as frail, vulnerable, and lacking in the degree of individual agency that they feel they need to manage everyday life and influence outcomes that they wish to affect (Gilleard & Higgs, 2010).

A final challenge that is likely to affect a person's well-being in old-old age, described in detail in an earlier chapter, is the loss of family and friends. With the absence of these long-term relationships, people can no longer share their history and memories, receive validation as to who they are and have been, and experience the same degree of companionship and pragmatic support that they were likely to have received in the past.

People tend to cope in one of two ways with this increasingly limited social network. They may realistically recognize that they are more on their own and do the best that they can to maintain the social network that they do have, or they may despair, anticipate that they are likely to become more and more isolated, and based on this expectation, withdraw, thereby reducing whatever socialization opportunities that exist still further (Johnson & Barer, 1993).

The following vignette illustrates several of the key ideas noted in the selective review of the literature:

His hemoglobin was again too low; this would be the fourth time this month that he would have to return to the hospital for a transfusion. Stanley, age 93, felt weak, tired, and weary. For almost 45 years, up until his mid-sixties, he had been the doctor – the one that others came to for help and the person they depended on. Now he was perpetually the patient, almost always having to depend on others. And instead of feeling the respect that he was used to, more and more, when he walked slowly and had difficulty getting up from a chair, he felt pitied, looked at as a frail, a struggling old man.

With his wife and all his close friends deceased, Stanley relied primarily on his oldest daughter to get him places and arrange for the aides he needed to look out for him when he was home. What mattered most to him now were his children and grandchildren. However crummy or depressed he felt on the inside, he wanted to act in ways that could serve as a model for how he hoped to be remembered by them.

Part two: Maintaining and enhancing well-being in old-old age

The following ideas and strategies can be used by clinicians if a person raises one or more of the following concerns during a clinical encounter.

Helping a person be as proactive and exert as much personal control as possible

When a person in old-old age mentions that they have nothing to look forward to and as a result, does not enact actions that might help them maintain their health and life satisfaction, a clinician can note that many people feel this way at this point in their life (Lennings, 2000). He or she can then explain that people who seem happier and more satisfied with life do not dwell on how life will be and instead focus primarily on the present; they try to maintain a sense of positivity by focusing on what they can do now and not the distant future (Carstensen et al., 1999). For example, they set health goals and make it more likely that they will ward off disease, lessen the risk of impaired health, and prevent further physical deterioration.

The clinician might also explain that people's sense of well-being is likely to be higher when they continue to exert effort to achieve these relatively short-term goals. And by doing so they demonstrate to themselves and others that they are still competent, able to exert personal control, and still committed to following the advice of the poet Dylan Thomas, who advised that in old age people should "not go gentle into that good night". When they do not go gently into the night, they are more likely to feel pride because they demonstrate that they are still as self-reliant as they can be and still an active decision-maker, exercising as much choice and control as possible, whenever they can (Atchley, 1997) and especially when they get affirmation from others that their self-sufficiency is recognized (Menninger, 1999).

The clinician can empathize with the increasing reality that with advancing age a person's ability to influence situations declines (Baltes & Baltes, 1990). The clinician can point out, however, that when people distinguish what they can influence and what they cannot, and choose to accept their lack of control and "go with the flow", their well-being is relatively higher (Chipperfield et al.,

2012). For example, when a person recognizes that they now have to depend on others to carry out many tasks, they are likely to maintain their self-worth, sense of autonomy, identity, and sense of engagement with life, especially if they still use their own core values to make choices and not passively let others make important decisions for them (Erikson, 1985; Brandstädter & Greve, 1994).

Setting realistic expectations

When talking about "looking forward", the clinician can mention that people are more likely to maintain a sense of well-being in old-old age if they set and accept realistic expectations – if they anticipate that they will be less able to change or affect many things they might wish to the degree that they would like to or were able to in the past (Tornstam, 1989). The clinician can explain that many people feel frustrated and self-critical at these times and their well-being is likely to be higher if they try to be accepting and self-compassionate – if they do not view what they can no longer do not as a weakness or a failure, but instead, as a reflection of the "season of life" they now occupy.

The clinician can also mention that a person is likely to have a greater sense of well-being if they do not continuously compare themselves to how they used to be, but rather judge themselves based on what is usual for most people when they are old-old; what others their age that they know are like; and especially, the degree to which they continue to exert effort to engage in activities that give them pleasure and satisfaction (Johnson & Barer, 1993).

Remaining active and social

When an elderly person describes feeling dissatisfied with their life, and has difficulty justifying why they should want to continue to live, for example, saying that they spend their day sitting alone, without speaking to anyone or participating in any social activities, the clinician can first review a typical day in the person's life from the time they get up till the time they go to sleep. In this way the clinician can better appreciate what the person does and does not do. If in fact the person is passive and isolated, the clinician can explain the importance of exerting effort to participate in physical and social activities (Herzog, Franks, Markus, & Holmberg, 1998) and highlight that it is difficult to not be despairing if they see their life as having little purpose or meaning (Erikson, 1963).

The clinician can note that when people are able to find ways to be active, their mood is likely to be higher; counter-intuitively, they are likely to feel less fatigued; they are more likely to experience a sense of pride; and they are more likely to see themselves as competent, purposeful, and productive (Herzog et al., 1998; Rowe & Kahn, 1998). They are also more likely to experience enjoyment (Palys & Little, 1983), especially if the activities that they select include contact with people that in the past they have felt close to (Lang & Carstensen, 1994; Rowe & Kahn, 1998).

If the person is open to suggestions, the clinician can also attempt to explore with the person social opportunities and resources in their community as well as suggest that a family member join the discussion and help plan.

Helping a person decide how best to view their age

When talking to a clinician, a person in old-old age may refer to their advanced years as a depressing, negative fact. If this was to happen, the clinician might mention that how a person views their age is likely to impact their sense of well-being. Thus, people tend to have a relatively higher degree of well-being if they can view the high number of years that they have lived in a positive light; if, for example, they can take pride in how their "good" genetic endowment and/or lifestyle has kept them alive for so long.

People are also likely to have relatively higher levels of well-being, the clinician can point out, if they attach a positive value to the knowledge that they have accumulated by living as long as they have and having the wealth of experiences that they did, especially if the person is able to find ways to share and have others appreciate this knowledge (Baltes & Staudinger, 2000; Ardelt, 2004; Fazio, 2010).

The importance of recognizing and savoring meaningful moments

Lastly, if a person seems "down in the dumps" and focuses primarily on what is negative about their life or about having as many functional limitations as they have, the clinician can mention that they may consider attempting to record in some fashion (i.e. by journaling or using a recording device) past or present moments, activities, and relationships that provide or have provided them with meaning and pleasure (Butler, 2002). When people are able to switch their attention from the negative aspects of their life towards what they appreciate and feel grateful for, they are found to be less distressed and relatively happier and satisfied (Wood, Froh, & Geraghty, 2010).

The following vignette illustrates several of the strategies that have been mentioned:

After the transfusion, Stanley's red blood count was still relatively low. He was advised to stay in the hospital till the next day to make sure that his hemoglobin levels were in an acceptable range. The following morning, the physician, who had been a former colleague of Stanley's, suggested that Stanley meet with the social worker, saying that Stanley seemed sad and unusually quiet the last few times that he had seen him. Stanley was open to the idea, gathered his things and went down to the social worker's office. After introducing herself, she explained that all she knew about Stanley was that he may be depressed. She asked if he could tell her if that in fact was the case, and if so, if he would describe in detail what he thought was causing him to be unhappy and dissatisfied.

Stanley hadn't really told anyone how awful he felt. He took a moment to gather his thoughts and then explained that recently he had not only felt physically exhausted but emotionally exhausted as well. He had always taken pride in his ability to work hard, exert tremendous effort, and persevere whenever he wanted to achieve a goal that was important to him. Lately, he kept wondering if there was a point to pushing himself anymore; and like the words to the famous song, "Que sera sera, whatever will be will be", most of the time he had little desire to do much of anything.

The social worker listened attentively and said that Stanley must feel extraordinarily worn out because of his anemia, and discouraged because the treatments seemed to last for only a short period of time before he needed another one. She wondered if he might be so preoccupied with how frustrating his situation was that he wasn't thinking about things in his life that could bring him satisfaction and pleasure. Stanley thought what she said was correct and realized that he had become more and more withdrawn. As a result, it was likely that he was reducing the chances of experiencing something positive even further.

The social worker also suggested that when Stanley felt strong enough he might try to see if he could act more like his prior self, and put out effort to achieve the goal of having satisfying moments. If he did, she said, he might again take pride in being the hard worker that he was used to being.

When Stanley got home from the hospital, he thought about his conversation with the social worker. He liked the idea of acting in ways that in the past made him proud of himself but knew that he would have to be very conscious as he did so of his current, very real health limitations. In thinking about how he might try to be like his "old self", Stanley went to get one of his favorite books, a memoir written by Sir William Osler, a physician that Stanley had emulated since the time he had begun medical school. Osler was the model of the physician that he had strived to be – a caring practitioner who really listened to his patients, and a person who stayed active throughout his life and pursued many interests. Stanley thought that, as in medical school, he would try to imitate his hero once again. He too would write a memoir, but unlike Osler, not try to publish it. Instead, he would give it to his children and grandchild so that they would have a record of who he was and know what had mattered most to him.

In addition to writing about his life, Stanley also thought that when he had enough energy, he would invite his children and grandson George to visit more regularly. When George, a first year medical student, did come to visit, he was curious about what it was like when Stanley had gone to medical school and asked many questions. After he left, Stanley realized how wonderful it felt to share the knowledge he had collected over many years, to have what he had shared be appreciated, and was looking forward to having future conversations with his grandson.

Summary

Significant differences exist in the needs, pressures, and circumstances people experience as they enter old-old age, differences that are likely to strongly affect their well-being. Given the variability in rates of aging, when defining the start of old-old age, it is important to consider biological and subjective or perceived age and not simply rely on chronological age as a start-point.

It is also important to recognize the psychological distinctions between young-old and old-old age. In young-old age people are likely to feel that they are relatively similar to the person they have always been, able to find ways to compensate for any limitations that they experience, can do many of the things that they have done in the past, and likely to still feel independent and efficacious. In contrast, in old-old age, people are likely to feel that they are no longer the same person that they were, in part, because they are now less able to overcome obstacles and carry out many of the tasks that they had previously valued, and in part, because they cannot rebound as well or as quickly from obstacles and setbacks. As a consequence, they are more likely to see themselves, and be seen by others, as dependent and less capable.

When speaking with a person who is in old-old age, a clinician needs to be alert to help the person cope with several challenges that are likely to arise and negatively affect their sense of well-being. These challenges include: becoming too preoccupied with the limited time a person in old-old age has remaining to live and difficulties in exerting personal control; feelings of dependency; difficulties in maintaining a positive self-image; and the need to cope with an increasing number of losses.

A clinician might explain that well-being in old-old age is likely to be relatively higher if people focus on the present and near future. By doing so a person is more likely to be motivated to exert effort, for example, to improve their health and be less frustrated and despairing. In addition, the clinician can point out the importance in old-old age of continuing to exercise choice – to try to be the "captain of their ship" as much as possible. Finally, the clinician might mention that people are more likely to maintain and enhance their sense of well-being if they appreciate the knowledge and valuable experiences that they have accumulated, particularly if they are able to share what they have learned with others.

Chapter 8

Three additional threats to a person's well-being in old-old age

Loneliness, a loss of purpose, and a feeling of mattering less

Part one: A selective review of the literature

A Loneliness

The older people are the more likely, as has been mentioned several times, they will experience multiple losses (de Vries & Johnson, 2002) and feel like a survivor who has outlived many of the individuals in their shrinking friendship and family social networks (Forster et al., 2018). As a consequence, in addition to being more selective with age as to who they want to socialize with, they are more likely to participate in fewer social activities (Carstensen, Isaacowitz, & Charles, 1999) and have an increasing number of friends and relatives with health impairments that limit the possibility of socializing. Therefore, in old-old age people are less likely to feel recognized and acknowledged and especially, less likely to have a sufficient number of confidantes (Victor, Scambler, Bowling, & Bond, 2005).

This expected decline in social interaction as people age is likely to result not only in feelings of social isolation but feelings of loneliness as well. While reported estimates of loneliness among older people vary a great deal, most studies find that between 30 to 40% of old-old people report feeling lonely and about 7% of respondents state that loneliness is a severe problem, especially after they have reached age 80 (Cacioppo, Grippo, London, Goosens, & Cacioppo, 2015; Tiilikainen & Seppanen, 2017).

Loneliness defined

Loneliness and social isolation are not synonymous (Bouwman, Aartsen, van Tilburg, & Stevens, 2016). While social isolation is typically defined as the objective lack of meaningful and sustained interactions with others (Chappell & Badger, 1989), loneliness is primarily considered to be a perception – a belief that a discrepancy exists between what a person desires to experience and what they feel they are actually experiencing in their social relationships (Cacioppo et al., 2015).

When a person is lonely, they are likely to compare their current social relationships to either past relationships, relationships that they hope to have, or relationships that they perceive others have. They then focus on the discrepancy that they believe exists between what they wish for and what they actually feel is present, and based on this judgment, experience such hurtful feeling as being separate, disconnected, empty, and rejected. In addition, what may seem counterintuitive is that people are especially likely to feel the pain of loneliness when they are in the presence of other people. The reason seems to be that the discrepancy between what a person wishes to feel and what they actually feel is more salient in this circumstance (Rook, 1984).

Further, when people are lonely, it is not just anyone that they tend to long for. Typically people long for a particular relationship – a specific one that they have had in the past, such as with a deceased spouse (Hartog, 1980), a friend they have lost touch with, or a fantasized person (Qualter et al., 2015).

Factors that influence the likelihood of experiencing loneliness

Early attachment experiences with caregivers are likely to affect both how frequently and intensely a person experiences loneliness. People are more likely to feel isolated and lonely as they age if they have had frequent separations from their primary caregivers early in life and have regularly felt disconnected from these primary sources of security. It is not only physical separations that can increase the risk of loneliness. Being psychologically separated can contribute as well. Thus, people are more likely to feel lonely as they get older if they have repeatedly experienced the absence or withdrawal of love, attention, and stimulation when they were a child (Hartog, 1980; Bowlby, 1960).

In old-old age, feelings of loneliness are especially likely to arise when people feel isolated or disconnected from others that they have felt attached to in the past, such as their children and spouse; a close social relationship ends due to death or physical separation; and a valued relationship ends following a profound misunderstanding or disagreement (Aartsen & Jylha, 2011; Hartog, 1980).

Loneliness and well-being

Experiencing loneliness over a relatively long period of time adversely affects both a person's physical and mental health. With regard to physical health, when people feel lonely for a prolonged period of time, they are at increased risk of experiencing cognitive decline, sleep disturbance, fatigue, and a high number of psychosomatic and physical symptoms (Bouwman et al., 2016; Theeke, 2009). They are also more likely to have a shorter life span compared to others who have relatively better social networks, in part because they have a less functional support system and less of a stress-buffering outlet that personal relationships can provide (Ellwardt, van Tilburg, Aartsen, Wittek, & Steverink, 2015).

With regard to mental health, chronic feelings of loneliness in late life increase the likelihood that a person will experience depression, low self-esteem, feelings of uselessness, and overall, result in a high level of distress (Saklofske & Yackulic, 1989; Aartsen & Jylha, 2011; Rokach, 2014).

B Doubts about mattering

As mentioned, in old-old age people are likely to participate in fewer activities and occupy fewer social roles. As a consequence, they are more likely to experience a loss of status and feel less recognized and appreciated by others; feel that fewer people pay attention to them and rely on them; and have fewer opportunities to feel that they are being truly seen and heard by others. In addition, again as mentioned, in old-old age people are more likely to be exposed to negative, devaluing stereotypes attached to "old people". The result is that late in life people are at increased risk of feeling that they do not matter as much as they did in the past or as much as they wish that they did (Froidevaux, Hirschi, & Wang, 2016).

"Mattering" defined

While the word "mattering" has many meanings, in the present context, it refers to being the focus of consideration or concern (Trumble, 2002). People tend to feel that they matter when they perceive that others view them as significant; are a recipient of the interest and attention of others; are depended on; and are convinced that their welfare concerns others. As with loneliness, a person's belief that they matter is not the result of an objective assessment; it too is a perception, a perception usually based on whether people important to them are demonstrating a sufficient degree of awareness of their needs and feelings and are influenced by their attitudes and actions (Dixon, 2007).

Therefore, mattering has several essential elements. A person feels that they are receiving a sufficient quality and quantity of attention from others; are important and useful to others; are a recipient of concern and support; believe that others appreciate the significance of events that are of concern to them (e.g. others will feel pride when the person makes a significant accomplishment or will feel upset when the person is upset); and are convinced that others pay attention not because of a personal benefit that they receive but care as an end in itself (Elliot, Kao, & Grant, 2004; Dixon, 2007).

People usually assess the degree to which they matter by making comparisons. They may compare how much attention they are getting with how much attention others are getting and if they conclude that they are getting a relatively smaller amount of attention than the other person is getting, feel they do not matter as much as they want to matter. They may also compare their situation to a social norm, for example, how many times a daughter calls them compared to how many times others in their social circle report getting calls from their children. If the amount is less, they may feel less significant than they want to feel. Lastly, they may compare the value that they feel they have now to another person with the value that they believe they had in the past (e.g. a mother now feels that she matters less because the daughter in the previous example had called her weekly in the past but now only calls her once every other week) (Mak & Marshall, 2004).

Mattering and well-being

The degree to which a person feels noticed, listened to, and useful strongly impacts their sense of well-being. When people feel that they matter they are more likely to have a sense that they belong and feel secure (Mak & Marshall, 2004); perceive themselves as valuable and have a relatively higher sense of self-esteem (Marshall, 2001); and experience a greater sense of global self-worth (Froidevaux et al., 2016).

When people feel they do not matter – when they feel that they are invisible, unimportant, and unappreciated, they are more likely to become depressed and feel alienated and marginal to others. As a result, in a self-fulfilling, damaging manner, they are at increased risk of becoming withdrawn, thereby making it even more likely that they will be less visible, noticed, and appreciated by others (Mak & Marshall, 2004).

C The loss of purpose

As mentioned in detail in Chapter 2, people are more likely to have a relatively higher sense of well-being if they are satisfied with their life – if they feel that what they have done and are doing is not only valuable to them but valuable to others as well (Baumeister, 1991). The degree of satisfaction that a person feels is not only influenced by the degree of clarity that they have about the value of what they are doing or have done but also by the degree to which they are able to apportion their time to achieve goals that they still believe are valuable.

Thus, in old-old age, if people are unable to identify and continue to work to achieve goals related to their life purpose, they no longer have a framework to organize and prioritize their time and make decisions as to how to allocate their personal resources (i.e. to decide what is worth spending money on and how much of their money they should spend) (Baltes, 1997; Baltes & Baltes, 1990; McKnight & Kashdan, 2009). Further, without valued goals, they are less likely to be motivated to initiate actions and persevere especially if obstacles arise (Folkman & Greer, 2000).

Purpose and well-being

Similar to the effects of loneliness, when a person experiences a loss of purpose, their physical health is likely to be negatively affected because they are less likely to engage in actions that might prolong their life. Thus, both men and women who felt that their life lacked purpose exercised less, exerted less effort to take care of their health, and engaged less in such preventative health actions as obtaining a cholesterol test or going for a colonoscopy (Holahan & Suzuki, 2006).

Comparing the effects of a loss of purpose in late life by gender, women who felt a lack of purpose were less likely to get a mammogram and men who felt a lack of purpose were less likely to get a prostate exam (Kim, Strecher, & Ryff, 2014). Therefore, for both men and women, failing to have and maintain a valued life purpose contributed to feeling there was less of a reason to exert effort to prolong their life, thereby substantially increasing their risk of mortality (Boyle, Barnes, Buchman, & Bennett, 2009).

In addition to the negative health consequences associated with a loss of purpose in late life, negative psychological consequences are evident as well, especially if the person is already depressed (Irving, Davis, & Colliuer, 2017). Thus, without a reason to live, a person is likely to be at a loss as to what to do to experience pleasure or satisfaction. If they attribute the reason for their loss of purpose to something they did or did not do (e.g. they didn't show sufficient interest in their grandchildren and now the grandchildren do not want to visit; they said hurtful things to the spouse of their son so they are invited over much less), the person is likely to feel what is missing from their life is their fault. They are then more likely to be self-critical, feel less worthy (Frankl, 1984; Irving et al., 2017), and in self-defeating fashion, even less likely to do things that might provide opportunities to feel useful or satisfied with their life (Froidevaux et al., 2016).

At times, the loss of a sense of purpose and a failure to identify goals that seem important or valuable may result in a person feeling that there is no justification or reason to continue to live and view the prospect of continuing to live as undesirable (Pinquart, 2002; Irving et al., 2017). Thus, without a valued goal to work towards, a goal that is perceived as necessary or valuable, a person is at risk of feeling that their life has been "completed" (van Wijngaarden, Leget, & Goossensen, 2015) or are indifferent as to whether or not they remain alive (Frankl, 1984). They might think, for example, that they would be better off if they no longer had to experience the ache of loneliness, anxiety about the unknowns that lie ahead, or frustration when they have to depend on others (van Wijngaarden et al., 2015).

The following vignette illustrates several of the key ideas noted in the selective review of the literature:

The clock read 3:12 a.m. Almost exactly the same time that she woke up yesterday. Her legs hurt and she assumed that was what woke her. The day stretched before her. Intimidating. She had no idea what she would do. The aide wasn't coming today and her children had come by briefly on the weekend. They wouldn't feel any obligation to come or call now for a few days.

As Dorothy, age 89, lay in bed, she couldn't shut off her mind. She thought she was a good mother who deserved some return for the sacrifices she had made. Yet, her children ignored her, seemed oblivious when she was upset, and criticized her when she complained and asked them to visit and call more. Instead of being sympathetic, they said she was always angry and demanding. With difficulty, she got out of bed, made a cup of coffee, sat at her usual spot by the end of the kitchen table, and went back to wondering how she came to be so excruciatingly alone.

Her father had died when she was 11, and her mother, a seamstress, had worked from early in the morning till late at night and maybe because of that was always bitter and critical. Dorothy remembered feeling lonely then too. She thought of her husband Phillip and began to cry. How much she missed him, even missed all the things that, when he was alive, had annoyed her. She had gotten married when she was 17, and once Phillip left the military, they had spent all their free time together up until his death about 10 years ago. They had three children – two girls and a boy. Her thoughts would always go to her first, her oldest, her nurse-daughter who had died of cancer when Dorothy was in her early sixties. Dorothy felt bad for thinking it but it seemed one more unfair thing that had happened to her, that the child who was the most loving, who was always willing to look out for her, was the one taken from her.

After her death she and Phillip had moved, far away from her oldest daughter's children, children she had partly raised, felt very close to, and now hardly ever got to see. Up until two weeks ago, even though it was so early, she might have called Shirley, her closest living friend, but Shirley had suffered a stroke, could not speak, and was now living in a long-term care facility.

Glancing at the clock, Dorothy saw that only an hour had gone by; it felt like a day. She felt restless and once more thought about her children. Why did she matter so little to them? Was she too angry and asking too much? The man in the next apartment was close to her age and, like her, had lost his spouse. He said his children checked on him every day, and on weekends brought the grandchildren to visit. She felt envious; she wanted someone to worry about her, to make her feel she was worth something, not simply a burden.

To stop thinking she tried to get up and turn on the television but couldn't; her hip hurt too much. She felt trapped and invisible and didn't see much point to living.

Part two: Strategies to cope with these three threats

The following ideas and strategies can be used by clinicians if a person raises concerns during a clinical encounter about loneliness, a loss of purpose, or a feeling of not mattering.

A Loneliness

The need to assess the person's motivation to change and ability to set realistic expectations

When a person complains about loneliness, the clinician needs to assess if the person is willing and able to exert effort to understand and change some of the factors that may be contributing (Bouwman et al., 2016), for example, to decide if they have the energy to engage in actions necessary to increase their contact with others. The clinician can mention that some people when lonely are passive and feel defeated, while others are active, self-reflective, and willing and able to see what they can do differently. If the person is willing to exert effort, the clinician can offer to help the person better understand why they feel as lonely as they do (Rokach, 2014; Fry & Debats, 2002).

As part of this discussion, the clinician can assist the person in distinguishing what they can change from what they cannot change, and while doing so identify aspects of themselves and their social life that they have to accept as "the way it is". For example, the clinician might point out that if a person's health greatly restricts the amount and type of social activities they are able to engage in, the person may have to accept that they are likely to remain somewhat isolated, or if the person's spouse, siblings, and close friends are no longer alive, they might have to accept that they will continue to feel somewhat lonely no matter how many social experiences they eventually are able to participate in.

If the person is motivated, the clinician can also try to help them set realistic expectations, for example, explaining that while a person may feel more "visible" and stimulated once they start socializing, especially initially, they are not likely to feel as important to others or as relied on as they did in their past, long-standing relationships. To further clarify what the person is now longing for, the clinician might ask the person to describe what they specifically enjoyed when with others and together assess the degree to which these elements are now realistically attainable. For example, after listening to a person describe things she valued when spending time with her spouse before he died, the clinician can point out that it seems reasonable to hope that she might again enjoy several of the elements that she mentioned, such as having deep conversations, laughing, or sharing everyday events.

Finally, the clinician can mention that it is also possible to be less lonely by changing one's attitudes. For example, a person may have ended several relationships with people that they had been close to because these people angered or disappointed them. As a result, they are now more isolated. The clinician might suggest that the person might want to evaluate what is relatively more important to them – holding a grudge and feeling empty and bored or being more tolerant and willing to overlook someone else's imperfections.

Helping the person evaluate their social skills

One especially important role a clinician can play when someone describes feelings of loneliness is to help assess if social skill difficulties are contributing. The clinician might review the quality and quantity of the person's past relationships as well as elicit examples of current social encounters to determine if the person's loneliness might, for example, be due to a failure to initiate social exchanges or take social risks; a tendency to be withdrawn and quiet when around others; or an inability to listen well when conversing with others.

If the person's social behavior does seem to be contributing to their social isolation, the clinician can use some of the recent encounters that the person described and employ the technique of mental simulation – a form of cognitive rehearsal and future-oriented planning – to visualize alternative social behaviors that the person might try to enact (Brier, 2015). For example, the clinician might help the person picture themselves initiating conversations rather than sitting quietly and only being an observer, or picture themselves as an attentive listener rather than as someone who primarily talks at other people.

If the person is open to trying out some of the ideas suggested, the clinician can propose having a follow-up. During the "review" the clinician might give the person feedback, based on what they have shared, as to whether the person seemed oversensitive; prone to misperceiving others' intentions; or inaccurately viewed themselves as not being accepted or responded to positively by others when what they described seemed actually to have gone well (Rook, 1984).

The clinician might also highlight the importance of being self-disclosing in order to counter feelings of loneliness – to explain that when people choose to share personal, important feelings and thoughts with another person, their loneliness tends to lessen, especially if they feel that what they have shared has been heard accurately and understood. When this occurs, a person is likely to feel "truly known" and experience a sense of connection (Jourard, 1971; Solano, Batten, & Patish, 1982).

Helping a person expand their social network

The clinician can explain that the most direct way a person can lessen their sense of social isolation is to expand their social network; for example, they might rekindle a past relationship that was positive but not maintained or identify opportunities where they could socialize and when in these situations be alert to the presence of people who they might want to get to know better. The clinician can point out that social situations with a recurring format (i.e., a class, a regularly scheduled meeting of an organization) are especially good for this purpose because by repeatedly seeing the same people, they are likely to get to know them more deeply.

The clinician can note that joining an organization in which members cooperatively work to achieve a shared goal (e.g. working to help feed, find housing, and legal assistance for immigrants) has been found to be especially helpful in reducing loneliness. This type of social experience often provides a person with the sense that they are now a member of a group and therefore "belong" (Weiss, 1973). In particular, religious or spiritual groups the clinician can mention, have been found to facilitate a sense of community and connection (Rokach, 2014).

Seeing value in solitude

Lastly, the clinician can note that some people choose to combat loneliness, not only by socializing to "fill" their sense of emptiness but also by seeking and engaging in solitary experiences that provide them with pleasure and stimulation, such as photography, art, or music. By engaging in such experiences, the clinician can explain the person is likely to switch their attention away from their unmet needs towards something they enjoy and can feel empowered because they are relying exclusively on themselves to feel fulfilled (Rook, 1984; Bouwman et al., 2016).

B Feelings of not mattering

When a person seems to be struggling with the feeling that they matter less to others, the clinician might first inquire as to what the person believes has changed to cause them to feel the way they do, and next help the person identify the people who they wish to matter to and the ways that they would judge whether they matter (e.g. if the other person pays attention to them, visits them, empathizes, is available when they need support). Lastly, the clinician can help the person consider if their perceptions about how they are being treated are accurate.

The clinician can note that the feeling of mattering is primarily a perception. As a consequence, sometimes a person may feel less upset about mattering less if they carefully examine whether there are extenuating circumstances to explain why someone is responding differently now compared to the past. For example, if the person states that they are upset about the lack of attention they are getting from a friend who they described as having a pain condition, the clinician might wonder if the friend may be acting less attentive because she is now depressed, preoccupied, and distracted by her pain. Similarly, if someone describes being hurt by a friend's lack of interest in getting together and while discussing the relationship has mentioned that the friend's spouse has become increasingly disabled, the clinician might wonder if the friend is less interested in getting together because of his wife's worsening condition that more and more requires his care.

The clinician might also point out the possibility that the person's perception about mattering less may be a function of changes in their social network rather than a function of changes in their value to others. The clinician can explain that as people age, more and more people they have known are likely to have either died or be less available because of an illness or a handicapping condition. Thus, although "crummy", it is usual for a person to have less contact and receive less interest from people that they have known earlier in their life (Pinquart, 2002; Charles & Carstensen, 2010).

The clinician can also mention that, as with loneliness, some people try to be active and cope while others remain passive and forlorn. If the person is willing to be active they can consider what might be the most effective way they can make requests of others; tell others more directly what they wish to receive from them; make more of an effort to take the initiative and keep in touch with others; be more self-disclosing when they talk to others; offer others assistance in the hope that what they give, they will receive; and be alert to the possibility that they are being overly sensitive and might work harder at being perspective-taking and considering the other person's thoughts, feelings, and life situation before concluding that they matter less.

Helping the person create new opportunities to matter

The clinician can also propose that the person might consider engaging in new experiences in which they could feel that they matter and might be recognized, appreciated, valued, and relied on. For example, they might volunteer and work cooperatively with others to assist a needy population (e.g. prepare meals alongside others to feed the homeless at a food kitchen). Many people who have done such "do-good" projects, the clinician can explain, have reported that they have felt more "visible" as a result because their efforts were acknowledged and appreciated, and others now depended on them, so that they felt they were still useful (Hansen, Aartsen, Slagsvold, & Deindl, 2018).

In addition to do-good projects, the clinician could mention that some people increase their sense of mattering by participating in an established, well thought-out, social movement (e.g. working to establish equal pay for women). When people choose to engage in a cause, the clinician can explain, they are more likely to feel that they matter because they have evidence that they are still "making a difference" and typically get feedback from others that they are.

C The loss of purpose

Transformative events

In late life, a clinician can explain, people who lost a sense of purpose may regain it through a transformative event, such as the serious illness of their adult child, or a political event that profoundly affects them, such as the election of an unpopular president. As a result of this life-changing event, the person acquires a meaningful goal to work towards, such as devoting themselves to their seriously ill child or working with others to elect a new president.

The clinician can point out that, more typically, when people regain their sense of purpose, they do so by being self-reflective and expending effort to identify or rediscover a goal that they come to find as valuable. A person might try to identify objectives they have worked towards in the past and found fulfilling; remember occasions they felt were highly significant and believed what they were doing mattered to them a great deal; or consider interests that were important and enjoyable to them earlier in their life but they either did not have the time or resources to pursue.

The clinician can mention that in surveys of people in late life, most people report that they find a sense of purpose by volunteering and artistic activities (Pinquart, 2002; Irving et al., 2017), seemingly because these types of activities often allow them to set goals and thus provides them with a sense of direction and a feeling of productivity (McKnight & Kashdan, 2009). Volunteering, in particular, the clinician can note has been found to strengthen a person's sense of meaning, self-worth, and life satisfaction, seemingly because when people volunteer they tend to feel that they are extending themselves for others in a truly "voluntary" fashion and are therefore doing something that is inherently "good" (Hansen et al., 2018).

The following vignette illustrates several of the strategies that have just been described:

During a routine visit with her internist, the doctor noticed how dejected Dorothy seemed. He suggested that she speak to a nurse located on the first floor of the same office building who was a certified geriatric counselor. Dorothy agreed, found the office, and set up an appointment for the following week.

When Dorothy greeted the counsellor, she felt comforted by her warm greeting. The counselor asked Dorothy to call her Sarah and suggested that Dorothy might start by telling her as much as she could about what was bothering her now, and what would be most important for Sarah to know about herself and her life. Dorothy began by describing her sleep. She said that it had always been bad but now it was awful. She said that she slept in short spurts throughout the night and whenever she woke she would immediately start to think about how lonely and angry she was. It didn't seem fair, she told Sarah – she had been a good mother and now was getting nothing back. It was as if she had already died and been forgotten.

Dorothy explained that she was especially upset with her children; instead of acting as if she had any importance, they made her feel like an annoying burden. As Dorothy talked, Sarah empathized and asked for specific examples of occasions when Dorothy felt that her children had let her down. Dorothy told how yesterday her daughter said she couldn't visit because she was going to help out and talk to veterans at a local veterans' center with a friend instead of coming over to visit and help her, and how her son, who owned a tech company, said he couldn't come this whole week to fix her computer because he was too busy with work even though his work was only a few miles from where she lived.

Sarah asked Dorothy if there were some people who she felt did care about her. Dorothy tearfully said that most of the people who had loved her and who she had talked to regularly were either dead, too sick to talk, or very far away. When asked to explain more, Dorothy said that her oldest daughter had died. She told Sarah that she had been a nurse like her and had three daughters that she knew cared about her but lived in another part of the country.

Sarah asked if Dorothy felt she had anything to look forward to. Dorothy said no and that getting through each empty day felt like torture. Lately she said she kept thinking that it would be better if she were no longer alive. Then she wouldn't have to feel so lonely.

Sarah told Dorothy that she could see how much pain she was in and that it seemed understandable because of all the empty time that she had, the losses that she experienced, and her physical discomfort. She also said that from the examples Dorothy gave, her children did seem to be acting in a hurtful, self-centered manner that would make anyone feel angry and let down. She then said that Dorothy also seemed so angry and wondered if her anger might be harming her health and possibly keeping people away who might want to be closer to her.

Sarah suggested that helping Dorothy be less angry might be something that they could work on together and also suggested that even though her granddaughters were far away, perhaps if she were more open about what she was feeling, they might be willing to have more contact with her. Lastly, Sarah said that Dorothy seemed bright and thoughtful and perhaps together they might be able to come up with ideas as to what Dorothy could do to fill her time and socialize.

Dorothy did what Sarah suggested. She called her granddaughter Joy, told her how she had been feeling, and to her delight, Joy said she would come to stay with her for several days the following week. In anticipation of the visit, Dorothy began tidying up the house and for the first time in a very long time, cooked. When the day of the visit finally arrived and she hugged her granddaughter, Dorothy burst into tears. She told her over the next few days how lonely she had been and how trapped and bored she felt.

After Dorothy went to bed, Joy called her two sisters, relayed what Dorothy had said, and together they agreed that they would each call on a specific day of the week, and in addition, on a rotating basis, come to visit for at least a day or two every few months. Joy told Dorothy about the plan and then asked her what it was like talking to Sarah. Dorothy said it was a relief. She was able to let out her feelings and thought that Sarah understood and actually cared about her.

After her granddaughter returned home, Dorothy thought more about Sarah's suggestion to get out of the apartment and socialize. One of the ideas they had discussed had to do with Dorothy's love of mahjong when she was younger. Dorothy had heard that several "seniors" played in the recreation room of her apartment complex once a week, decided to give it a try, and in fact enjoyed the game as well as the conversation very much. Encouraged, she was open to trying another idea that Sarah had suggested. She volunteered once a week to help at a Meals on Wheels, sitting alongside others wrapping the food that would be delivered to needy seniors.

Over time, Dorothy felt less bored and lonely. She now had a calendar with events to look forward to and people she was getting to know better and better. And for the first time in a very long time, was feeling less impatient and irritable.

Summary

As people approach old-old age, they are likely to have outlived many of the people that they have cared about and who have cared about them; feel less physically capable and healthy; and participate less in activities and social roles that have both provided them with a sense of belonging and set of goals. As a result, they are at risk of experiencing three threats to their well-being – loneliness, a feeling that they matter less to others, and a loss of purpose. Each of these threats, when realized, can have a deleterious effect on both their physical and mental well-being.

To counter these risks, a clinician can encourage the person to be self-aware and clarify what they feel is missing and desirable; assess if they are sufficiently motivated to put out effort to seek substitutes for what they feel has been lost; and while doing so, be realistic and adaptable and accept what they discover as satisfying even if it falls short of their ideal wishes or past experiences.

The clinician can also note that being socially active and joining social networks where they can take on cooperative, meaningful roles, especially roles that include helping others, could be especially valuable in decreasing loneliness, increasing feelings of mattering, and reigniting a sense of purpose. Lastly, the clinician can mention that people are more likely to manage these threats to their well-being if they are "transparent" when with others and tell others what they desire and feel.

Chapter 9

Decline, imminent death, and well-being

Part one: A selective review of the literature

An inevitable, progressive, biological decline

Worldwide, the number of very old people, people aged 80 years and older, is projected to increase dramatically from 125 million in 2015 to 202 million in 2030 (United Nations, 2015). These very old people who will live into their mid- and late eighties and nineties are likely to experience an irreversible and progressive decline in their functional abilities (e.g. in their ability to see, hear, move, and lift) and cognitive abilities (Isaacowitz & Smith, 2003), develop one or more functional impairments and chronic illnesses (e.g. angina, osteoporosis, spinal stenosis), experience chronic pain, and have multiple health co-morbidities (Young, Frick, & Phelan, 2009). To illustrate, 72% of 276 Danish centenarians were found to have cardiovascular disease, 54% osteoarthritis, and 41% dementia; all but one had between 4 and 5 illnesses on average (Andersen-Ranberg, Schroll, & Jeune, 2001).

There is also likely to be a parallel decline in personal resources needed to cope with the health problems that are present. Thus, the oldest old are less likely to be able to counterbalance the negative health changes that are occurring, or develop effective compensations and accommodations to cope with these problems (Rothermund & Brandstädter, 2003).

The result – an increasingly restricted life defined primarily by diminishing health

Thus, in very late life as a person experiences an increasing amount of physical discomfort and has less capacity to cope, two key markers of well-being are likely to decline – life is likely to be less pleasurable and less satisfying (Smith, Borcheit, Maier, & Jopp, 2002). In addition, a person is less likely to feel adequate and like the person they were in the past. Given the need to maintain a variety of medical treatment regimens and appointments, in very old age, in addition, the person is likely to define themselves by their health difficulties and plan and organize their time based on their health needs (Charmaz, 1983; Nekolaichuk & Bruera, 1998).

People at this stage are also likely to experience a heightened sense of uncertainty. They tend to be highly aware that their health will continue to decline but do not know when the next significant decrement in their health will occur; the degree or specific form that it will take; or how these anticipated health changes will impact and further restrict their ability to function. Thus, in very old age, people can look forward only tentatively. They tend to be very cognizant of the fact that any plans that they make, especially plans that extend somewhat into the future, may not actually come to be. Further, because of their uncertainty, anticipation of bad health days, and fears about travelling far from home, they increasingly restrict what they do and where they go (Charmaz, 1983).

A sense of sorrow

Very late in life, a sense of loss is likely also likely to be frequently present. Because of the need to depend on others a great deal, a person may grieve for what they can no longer do as well as grieve for the experiences that they can no longer participate in, for what will no longer be possible to see and know, and for the lack of support and comfort of family and friends that they had in the past. They may also feel self-critical and guilty for being a burden – a person who now requires a great deal of support from others, yet is unable to reciprocate (Smith et al., 2002; Molton & Jensen, 2010).

Imminent death: The ultimate challenge to a person's well-being

As a very old person's health continues to decline, they may be told that their death is imminent. When this occurs, in addition to whatever physical discomfort they may be experiencing, their well-being is likely to be further challenged by a sense of terror as they contemplate the possibility of non-existence or nothingness (Becker, 1973). Especially initially, they are likely to feel overwhelmed and unable to take in such frightening images as being separate from everyone and everything that they have known, unable to move, and gradually disintegrating (Lifton, 1973).

People tend to cope with this often overwhelming fear by vacillating back and forth between denying the reality of what they have been told, fighting against the accuracy of the information, feeling hopeless and despairing, and accepting what they imagine is in store (Sand, Olsson, & Strang, 2009). Individuals who are able to maintain a sense of agency, act with dignity, and not withdraw from others are found to be better able at this time to maintain a sense of equanimity (Chochinov, 2003).

More specifically, people are relatively less distressed towards the end of their life if they are as functionally independent as possible; actively participate in their care; expect, and if necessary, demand that they be treated empathically and respectfully especially on occasions where they cannot be independent; insist that others listen and treat what they have to say as if it has value; are viewed as an individual rather than as a generic "someone" occupying the role of a patient at the end of their life; are given assurance that their personal affairs will be respected and handled (e.g. that people have read and will follow their personal will and final end-of-life instructions); and, when desired, have their need for personal space and privacy respected (Chochinov, 2003).

The need for a framework to provide meaning, connection, and dignity

As discussed in prior chapters, a person's well-being is likely to be relatively higher if they can identify a meaning or purpose – a belief system that helps them view their existence as having value and provides them with ideas and images to lessen their terror as they anticipate what will occur after they die (Taylor, 1983; Sand et al., 2009). A person's well-being is especially likely to be relatively higher if the explanatory framework provides reassurance that they will continue to exist in some form after their physical death (Lifton, 1976).

Two other factors likely to support a person's well-being when death is imminent is the degree to which a person feels connected to others and the degree to which he or she is able to maintain their dignity. Thus, as a person anticipates being separated from themselves (i.e. their conscious mind) and the people who have mattered to them, feeling close to, cared about, and supported by others is likely to allay their separation anxiety and allow them to feel less alone and lonely (Yalom, 2008; Boston, Bruce, & Schreiber, 2011).

With regard to maintaining dignity, a person's well-being is likely to be relatively higher at this stage if they exert effort to be how they aspire to be and how they wish to be remembered. When a person consciously attempts to maintain their self-respect and self-esteem, they are more likely to experience a sense of agency and resist the urge to withdraw, seemingly because their attention is directed towards a valued goal and away from the dread of death and lack of personal control (Chochinov, Hack, McClement, Kristjanson, & Harlos, 2002).

The role and value of hope and goals

When a person is given a terminal diagnosis. their view of time is likely to be powerfully affected. They are now excruciatingly aware that they have only an uncertain, very limited period of time to live, instead of as in the past, especially when they were young, an infinite, "timeless future" (Cassell, 1976). A person's anxiety is likely to be relatively lower if they have hope that in the time they do have, they can achieve important, short-term, realistically attainable goals.

Based on studies of patients in palliative care, the end of life hopes that people typically select include: controlling their physical symptoms and pain; maintaining their sense of self-respect and self-worth; engaging in actualizing experiences (e.g. experiences that involve art or nature); participating in a specific event (e.g. a child's wedding); and interacting as much as possible with specific people whom they feel especially close to (Clayton, Butow, Arnold, & Paterson, 2005).

By having and working to realize such goals and having a "positive" to focus on, a person's self-esteem is likely to be relatively higher. The person can take pride in remaining as active and goal-directed as possible, being a positive model for the people they care about, and providing them with valuable life lessons (Clayton et al., 2005).

The following vignette illustrates several of the key ideas noted in the selective review of the literature:

For the last three years Aaron, age 76, had been struggling with heart problems. At first he was easily fatigued and short of breath yet could do most of the things that he had always done. Over time, however, even when he exerted himself only a little bit, he would feel weak and breathless. His cardiologist told him that he had congestive heart failure, prescribed medications, and regularly monitored his condition. Yet nothing seemed to help. Aaron was able to do less and less. Instead of being the independent caretaker that he had always been, he now had to depend on others and spend too much time in doctor's offices, surrounded by other sick, older people.

This past week Aaron had felt much worse. He had palpitations, several episodes of chest pain, couldn't stop coughing, and his ankles were swollen. Frightened, instead of waiting for his next scheduled appointment, Aaron called the doctor's nurse. He told her what was going on and was given an appointment for later that same day. The doctor, accompanied by a cardiology fellow, listened to Aaron's concerns. After doing a physical exam, the doctor told Aaron that his condition was significantly worse and he was now considered "Class IV". Unfortunately, he said, there is nothing that can be done to slow the progression of the illness. The cardiology fellow, while very attentive, remained silent.

Aaron couldn't fully take in what was being said. He felt a pressure at the top of his head and at the same time, detached, as if he were watching someone else doing what he was doing. He realized that the doctor was not saying what Aaron could expect going forward. He was not saying how long he had to live or how he would die. When Aaron asked, the doctor only said that the time Aaron had left to live would likely be relatively short and that the cause of his death would likely be Aaron's heart eventually failing.

The doctor then asked Aaron if he was as stoic as he appeared. Aaron paused, thought, and said, "I don't feel stoic at all; I am numb yet underneath feel an immense, profound sadness for the things that my children and grandchildren will do that I won't be able to see." While the doctor seemed to hear Aaron's words, he made no comment. He simply turned to leave, saying as he did, that he would see Aaron next week at the already-scheduled appointment time.

After the doctor left, the cardiology fellow spoke for the first time. He told Aaron that to hear what Aaron had just heard must be overwhelming and terrifying. The fellow went on to say that if Aaron wanted, he would be glad to meet with him to help him sort out his thoughts and feelings. Aaron thanked him and said he would call to set up an appointment.

Once home, Aaron thought about what he had been told. He was struck by what he felt was certain and uncertain. He felt certain that he would die in a relatively short time and uncertain just what a short time meant. He also felt certain that his heart would fail and uncertain as to what exactly would happen when it did. And, at the moment, he definitely didn't feel stoic; he felt very scared.

Unlike his father and siblings, Aaron had never been religious. He now wished that he could be like them and have a ready-made storyline about what would happen after he died, one that would provide him with comfort and replace the void that he pictured. He wished he could believe, like his brothers, that after death you enter a heaven and there is a benevolent god waiting to take care of you. Aaron was not sure what he could imagine that would provide some solace. He did know that he would feel better if he could believe that there was something next, rather than nothing, and that he would live on in some way and not simply stop existing.

Part two: Strategies to maintain well-being in the presence of our declining health and imminent death

The following ideas and strategies can be used by clinicians if a person raises one or more of the following concerns.

Helping the person face their terror

When a person is experiencing declining health and actively considering the prospect of death, a clinician can provide an invaluable and difficult service by encouraging the person to speak about their thoughts and feelings. These conversations are likely to be extremely challenging for a clinician because it is difficult both to experience another person's pain and suffering, and the anxiety attached to a foreshadowing of the clinician's own decline and death. Yet by participating in these conversations, the clinician is providing the person something that is essential – a human connection that can lessen the person's fears about being separate from all that they have known and an opportunity for catharsis.

By carefully listening, clarifying, validating, and offering empathy and compassion, the clinician can help the person express their needs, fears, wants, final wishes, and end of life preferences. As a result, they are likely to be better able to anticipate, plan, and problem-solve in regard to how they will deal with the challenges that they are occurring, and likely to experience an increase in their sense of personal control and ability to regulate their actions and emotions (Ouwehand, de Ridder, & Bensing, 2007).

During these discussions, the clinician can also help the person develop a detailed description, or set of guidelines, as to how they wish to act as they approach the end of their life. These guidelines can provide the person with "targets" that they can aim for that can help them divert their attention away from their fears and towards a set of aspired goals. Not only can these goals serve as diversions, they can also be a source of satisfaction, a way the person can take pride in demonstrating that he or she is the the person they wish to be and that they are shaping how they hope to be remembered.

To help the person develop these guidelines, the clinician can describe the typical aspirations of others when in the same situation. People usually aspire to identify and demonstrate specific behaviors that they would be proud of (e.g. being assertive when they were not heard); be like someone they admired when that person was facing a serious health crisis or approaching the end of their life (e.g. a parent, famous individual); model values that are especially important to them (e.g. acting with calmness, being kind, being perspective-taking even when suffering); or, be how they have always been in the past (e.g. asking questions, being assertive) (Brandstädter, 1989). The clinician can note that people are more likely to experience a relatively higher level of well-being when death seems relatively near if they exert effort to the extent that they can to maintain as many of their regular activities and routines that they feel have previously defined them (e.g. reading, photography). When they do, they are more likely to feel the positive feeling linked to a sense of continuity with their past (Charmaz, 1983; Rowe & Kahn, 1997).

Finally the clinician can point out that it is important to continue to plan to do things that in the past have provided positive expectations, pleasure, and satisfaction; for example, they might schedule and then look forward to times when they can have intimate, "deep" conversations with certain people, or attend a special occasion of a loved one (e.g. a son's upcoming birthday celebration), even if it is unclear that they will actually be able to do so.

Maintaining autonomy and a sense of agency

The clinician can explain that feeling autonomous and exercising a sense of agency are key elements of well-being. Thus, if the person chooses, in Dylan Thomas's words, not to "go gentle into that good night" (Erikson, 1985; Brandstädter & Greve, 1994), and instead, is an active decision-maker, they are likely to feel a greater degree of personal control and as a result, be less anxious (Atchley, 1997; Montross et al., 2006). The clinician can note that it is especially important to exercise personal control in regard to health decisions; for example, to tell their health care providers how much they want to know about their medical status (e.g. from very little to everything), how they want the information to be presented (e.g. with "sugarcoating" or without any "sugarcoating"), and what their end of life preferences are (e.g. avoiding unnecessary procedures, minimizing pain).

The clinician, in addition, can point out that it is also important for the person to feel empowered to change these preferences as their health continues to decline. For example, they may at one point feel they need to rely on illusions for comfort and want to know less and at another point, may want to know more so they can have a better sense of what is coming and plan.

Identifying a meaning framework

As previously detailed, the clinician can tell the person that identifying and articulating a meaning framework, or set of beliefs, can help them accept what they can no longer control and to create an expectation of what lies ahead (Crowther, Parker, Achenbaum, Larimore, & Koenig, 2002). Thus, when someone is able to identify and "buy into" a meaning framework, they tend to reduce their dread of the unknown and struggle less with the task of having to counter the dread of "nothing" (Kirkegaard, 1957).

Some people, the clinician can mention, instead of seeking a formal, organized set of beliefs to allay their anxiety, try to experience a sense of connection between themselves and another person, or themselves and all living things. If the idea of connectedness or transcendence seems of interest, the clinician can explain that proponents of this approach might imagine they are letting go of their personal boundaries and merging with, or flowing into, something larger and more enduring than themselves by focusing their attention on aspects of nature; an object attached to spirituality such as a religious symbol; or imagining they are interacting in a caring way with a deceased family member or friend who they have felt especially close to (Lifton, 1973; Frankl, 1984).

The clinician can further explain that the beliefs a person chooses to cope do not need to be realistic. Rational or irrational, thoughts about what is to come can be considered to be valuable to the extent that they bring comfort and decrease uncertainty (Yalom, 1980; Taylor, 1983; Kastenbaum, 2009).

Finally, the clinician can mention that if the person can identify what they feel matters most to them, their well-being is also likely to be relatively higher. When they do, they create opportunities to focus their energy during the time they have remaining. In addition, they are more likely to use the time they have to look back at their life and make salient and savor what they have deemed as extra important (e.g. how they have dealt effectively with adversity; occasions when they especially felt loved).

Clarifying how a person wishes to be remembered

The clinician can point out that most people desire to live on and be remembered and valued as they approach the end of their life. Towards this end, the clinician can suggest that the person consider telling those who matter to them (even if they have told them before) how and why they matter; what about their relationship has been most valuable; the particular moments that have been especially meaningful and precious; and their wished-for, future hopes for the person.

The clinician can also point out that people are found to be especially likely to gain satisfaction when sharing these thoughts if they dictate or write them out. By doing so, they produce a concrete and enduring record of what they want the person to remember (Chochinov, 2003). Unlike when a person writes a life review, described earlier, what is written in this context is selective, narrowly focused, and exclusively addresses what the person feels defines them and is important in the relationship with the person who they are sharing their thoughts and feelings with.

Staying connected

The clinician can explain that towards the very end of a person's life, they are likely to be less anxious and feel less alone if they do not withdraw and instead be as close to others as possible. The clinician can also mention that if the person has a pet, their anxiety is likely to be relatively lower if they are able to keep their pet nearby (Sand et al., 2009).

The following vignette illustrates several of the strategies that have been mentioned:

Two days later Aaron met with the Cardiology Fellow. The Fellow told him that he could forget titles if he wanted and just use his first name, Ernie. Aaron told Ernie that he had thought a great deal about his last visit with the cardiologist – how disappointed he was by the doctor's behavior; how the doctor had chosen to ask him about his feelings and yet, when given an answer, not only did he not show any compassion, he simply ignored what Aaron had said.

Ernie said that he was sorry that Aaron had been so upset and agreed that the doctor did not seem to recognize or respond in an appropriate way. He told Aaron that while the doctor was not known generally as having a wonderful bedside manner, the fact that he had lost his wife about 8 months ago might have contributed; even though it is professionally required, the doctor may still have found it too hard to directly discuss issues related to death and dying.

Aaron was comforted by Ernie's direct and caring manner. He told Ernie how these days he was always short of breath and exhausted whenever he attempted any type of physical activity; how his life had become more and more restricted, and how, for most of the day, he would just sit in his favorite chair staring at the forest behind his house.

Aaron went on to describe how he felt that the shock had worn off a little bit. He now felt mostly sad and scared. He said he wasn't quite sure what he was sad about but felt as if he were in mourning – that soon he would no longer being able to think, feel, and hear his inner voice, no longer be connected to his children and grandchildren, and no longer know about their lives. Aaron said that he did know what he was scared about – he was frightened of the unknown, of not being able picture how he would actually die or what would happen afterwards.

Ernie listened quietly, periodically asking follow-up questions to be sure that he understood. He told Aaron that many patients cope with the uncertainty of what lies ahead by developing a script, like in the movie Heaven Can Wait. *Included in the script are their hopes for something they imagine would be comforting. Ernie also mentioned that most people specifically want to come up with ways that they might continue to exist past their physical death. Some, he said, imagine that after they die and disintegrate, their molecules will reform into another type of living matter. Most people, however, hope that they will live on by being remembered by those who they have cared about. Ernie said that with regard to how Aaron's death was likely to arrive, most likely his heart would get weaker and weaker and eventually, like a clock when the spring finally unwinds, would simply stop; or Aaron would have an electrical problem, experience a short circuit, and then his heart would fail. Ernie reassured him that in either circumstance, with the aid of medications, he would not suffer. Ernie also said that the people who seemed most calm at the end of their life appeared as if they accepted their coming death and viewed it as the way it is; they didn't seem to struggle or protest. Instead they seemed to be able to relax and flow into whatever was coming next.*

Over the following weeks, as Ernie suggested, Aaron tried to picture what would happen after he died. He vacillated between two ideas. In one, he imagined being reunited with his mother, however unlikely that really was, and visualized in detail her face and her voice as she soothed and reassured him. In the other, he pictured that after death his remains would merge with the particles of all other living things in the universe and he would become some unknown other life form.

Remembering Ernie's comments about the importance of sharing what he felt with those he cared about, even though he felt exhausted, Aaron pushed himself to engage in conversations with his family. He told them once more what he considered to be the significant moments in his life and what he was particularly grateful for, proud of, and cherished most.

And in keeping with Ernie's idea of influencing how he wanted to be remembered, Aaron made an effort to not complain. He tried to be a loving listener and told about the life lessons that he thought were important, such as the importance of insisting on being treated respectfully by others and in being in charge of whatever choices have to be made.

Summary

If people live to a very old age, they are likely to experience a progressive decline in both their health and personal resources. A clinician can highlight that people often struggle between accepting what has changed or continue to try, often at this point without success, to compensate for the deficits that now exist. More and more of a person's time is now spent following medical regimens and seeing physicians to manage the impairments and illnesses that are present. It is more difficult to maintain a sense of well-being therefore due to the increasing presence of pain and discomfort; the greater degree of restriction in activities and social roles; and the challenges that are likely to be present in maintaining their identity and independence.

A clinician can highlight that during very old age most people are challenged by a sense of uncertainty. They know that their health will continue to decline but do not know the rate of decline or the particular form that the decline will take. As a result, they are likely to feel anxious as they anticipate the unknowns that lie ahead; sad as they grieve for what they can no longer do or be; experience an ever increasing reduction in their social network; and think about what in the future they will be unable to see and experience.

If a person learns that their death is in the relatively near future, a clinician can empathize with the feeling of terror that the person is likely to experience, especially as they contemplate the idea of non-existence. The clinician can point out that identifying a belief system might bring comfort by helping to create an image of what happens at and after death and in identifying and appreciating what they believe has been valuable about their life. The clinician can also encourage the person to set concrete, realistic goals that might divert their attention away from their fears and bring them pleasure and satisfaction in the time that they do have remaining.

Finally, in the face of a person's declining health and imminent death, the clinician can help the person set attainable aspirations and standards to guide how they wish to act in order to facilitate control and pride; create opportunities to experience moments of pleasure and satisfaction; be a self-advocate, especially in regard to their medical care; preserve their identity, in part by maintaining former routines and activities as much as they can; define how they wish to be remembered so that they can experience pride and satisfaction as they demonstrate these behaviors, and be as connected as possible to the people who matter to them.

Chapter 10

Summary and synthesis

The key ideas in regard to aging and well-being that have been presented will first be summarized, followed by a description of a set of factors that seem especially important in order to experience well-being when older.

Well-being and aging

Key literature-based findings

Psychological well-being is composed of two main elements – people experience a sense of well-being either when they experience pleasure and infrequently experience negative emotions, and feel self-actualized and see their life as satisfying, valuable, and purposeful (Diener, Suh, Lucas & Smith, 1999; Feeney & Collins, 2015). Seven sets of "ingredients" were said to play an especially important role in determining how likely it is that a person will experience well-being as they age. These ingredients include: an articulated set of life purposes; the presence of regularly occurring occasions in which a person feels pleasure and positivity; participating in close, supportive relationships; possessing an adequate level of self-esteem; experiencing personal control; and continuing to engage in activities that facilitate personal growth.

When people express concerns as they age that challenge their ability to experience these aspects of well-being, clinicians can suggest a variety of strategies to help manage what the person is experiencing as an obstacle or finding challenging. These strategies include helping a person to identify, articulate and continuously update their life purpose(s); carefully select and "optimize" the activities that they choose to engage in; be aware of what they appreciate and are grateful for; question and learn from their regrets; maintain and strengthen close, supportive relationships, especially longstanding ones; preserve their identity and self-esteem and note what is continuous about their life that they are proud of; exert personal control while concurrently noting and accepting a decreasing ability to influence events; and, lastly, seek and engage in novel intellectual, aesthetic, and physical activities in order to experience personal growth.

While it seems reasonable to expect that a person's level of well-being will decrease as they get older as their cognitive and physical abilities decline and their awareness and anxiety about mortality increases, the opposite is often true. With age many people seem able to maintain a relatively high level of well-being (Jeste et al., 2013). They seem to experience fewer negative emotions and are more self-accepting. Specifically, as people get older they seem better able to focus on and prioritize what is satisfying in the present and near future relative to the distant future; have greater emotional control and are less reactive when upsetting events occur; and are less self-critical and able to view their past accomplishments and failures in a balanced manner. As a result, they are more realistic in their appraisal of their strengths and limitations, less concerned about the judgments of others, and less likely to compete or compare themselves to others. Finally, they are more tolerant of ambiguity and uncertainty (Carstensen, 2006; Jeste & Oswald, 2014).

Social support is found to be essential in order for people to experience an adequate level of well-being as they get older (Ryff, 1995; Rowe & Kahn, 1998; Feeney & Collins, 2015). Long term relationships can be considered a protective "convoy" that "encircles" a person and makes it less likely that they will experience negative emotions, and more likely that they will experience security, comfort, practical assistance, and validation. As a result, people who have social support are more likely to feel valued and valuable and receive affirmation that they are still the same person that they were in the past.

Yet, as a person gets older, their social network is likely to shrink as more and more of their friends and family members either die or have health problems that limit their ability to socialize (Rook & Charles, 2017). In addition, with age people are likely to become more selective in who they want to socialize with and they are more likely to desire to spend time with friends they have known for long periods of time, which further reduce their social network (Lang & Carstensen, 1994). To help counter the increased risk of social isolation, a clinician might regularly inquire about how an older person is filling their time and specifically, the nature and frequency of their social activities.

Key strategies

When a person consults a healthcare professional and describes concerns that seem to be threatening their sense of well-being, the clinician can help the person clarify what they wish to achieve or experience at this point in their life that might allow them to feel that their life is purposeful and worthwhile, a feeling considered by many scholars to be fundamental to human flourishing and subjective well-being (Steptoe & Fancourt, 2019). The clinician might explain that when a person is aware of what they want to experience and achieve – their desired endpoint or "destination" – they are more likely to achieve it, in part because they now have a direction and a rationale or framework to support or justify their actions and a set of standards to help maintain their focus and sustain their motivation. They also have a guideline they can use to alter their actions and level of effort when needed (Hill & Turiano, 2014; Steptoe & Fancourt, 2019).

In addition, by having clarity about "what matters", a person is better able to allocate their personal resources – their time, money, and effort – to achieve goals and is more likely to be aware of when they are successful (Steptoe & Fancourt, 2019). As a consequence, they are more likely to be aware of occasions on which they feel proud and efficacious and experience pleasure and satisfaction (McKnight & Kashdan, 2009).

Mortality: The primary concern as people age

Key literature-based findings

As people get older and consult with healthcare professionals about their physical deterioration, illnesses, and often, multiple chronic conditions, the issue of mortality is likely to be either in the foreground or the background of their mind (Becker, 1973; Greenberg, Solomon, & Pyszcynski, 1997). They are likely to convey anxiety as well as sadness as they consider both dying and death (Kastenbaum, 2009). A clinician can provide a forum for the person to express what are often private thoughts and can explain that most people when older are concerned about mortality and come to view time as an increasingly scarce resource.

The clinician can further explain that, in particular, people have difficulty managing uncertainty. They of course know that ultimately they will die but feel anxious because they do not know exactly how or when death will arrive, what the experience will be like when it does, and what will happen afterwards (Pyzscynski et al., 1996). Adding to a person's sense of uncertainty and anxiety, the clinician can point out, is a decline with age in the degree of personal control that inevitably occurs, which results in an increased need to depend on others; the possibility of suffering when dying; and lastly, doubts about whether they will be able to cope adequately with what is to come (Baars, 2017a).

Key strategies

To help allay concerns about mortality, a clinician might explain that most people can manage their fear of non-existence by seeking or endorsing a set of beliefs that allows them to anticipate what happens when people die and afterwards and which provides them with rules and rituals (i.e. religious practices) to instill a sense of control and predictability (Greenberg et al., 1997). By ascribing to and enacting these beliefs, the clinician can point out that people are less uncertain about the unknowns that are ahead. For example, if a person subscribes to the idea of an afterlife, they are likely to be relatively less anxious because they can now anticipate and imagine what is to happen after their biological ending.

A clinician can also mention that many scholars believe that, at the core of mortality anxiety, is the fear of non-existence (Becker, 1973). Therefore, in addition to beliefs about an afterlife, the clinician might point out that people may feel less anxious if they can ascribe to the notion that they will continue to "live on", either as noted, because there is an afterlife, or indirectly or symbolically after their physical death, for example, by being remembered by their children and grandchildren or by people remembering and valuing something that they have created (e.g. a book or painting) (Case, Fitness, Cairns, & Stevenson , 2004).

Finally, the clinician can mention that some people do not try to "buy into" an organized belief system but instead try to manage their mortality anxiety by realism and acceptance – by viewing death as an inevitable, natural aspect of life, one that can be considered as similar to the "known" state that existed prior to their birth. Thus, they try to keep to the wisdom expressed in the song, "Que Sera Sera" – "whatever will be, will be; the future's not ours to see".

Following retirement and the loss of significant others: Maintaining a sense of self-continuity

Key literature-based findings

After such major life transitions as retirement or the loss of a significant relationship, a person may say during a clinical encounter that they no longer "feel themselves". A clinician can explain that it is usual for people to experience identity confusion following significant transformative events, after which they cease engaging in familiar activities, roles, and routines. The clinician can point out that most people are motivated as a result to feel that, in essential ways, they are still the same person after a significant change so that they can feel stable and grounded (Dunkel & Worsley, 2016). In addition, the clinician can also point out that, after the loss of familiar experiences and relationships that have linked the person's past and present, many people also feel sorrow and worry that valued parts of themselves may now be lost and never recovered (Schafer & Shipee, 2010).

Compounding this threat to a person's sense of self-continuity with age, the clinician can mention, is the likelihood of an increasing number of deaths of people who the person has known and who have known him or her (de Vries & Johnson, 2002). As a result, people increasingly lose a source of feedback and validation that has helped them affirm their identity and has linked them to their personal histories (Forster et al., 2018).

Key strategies

To help a person maintain their sense of identity, especially in the period immediately following a major life transition, the clinician can highlight the importance of creating a set of routines or life structure, even if only temporary, to provide order and predictability while the person "catches up" with the changes that have occurred. In addition, the clinician can explain that trying to focus on what matters to them at the moment, a life purpose, may help them feel that they have a set of goals and a direction to guide their choices, similar to how a mariner might use a compass to steer.

If the person ruminates a great deal about what they feel is now missing or lost from their life, the clinician can note that people tend to feel better following a life transition if they not only focus on what is missing or lost, but also focus on, remember, and savor the positives that they value and believe have enriched their lives. Especially after the death of someone particularly significant to them, the clinician can explain it is helpful to focus on the "continuing bond" that they still have with the person even though they are no longer physically present (Klass, Silverman, & Nickman, 1996), as well as on the life lessons that they have learned as a result of this relationship. By focusing on these positives, the clinician can explain, they are more likely to experience a greater sense of well-being (Seligman, 2002) and a link to their past (Klass et al., 1996).

The clinician can also mention that people experience a sense of self-continuity not only from their personal identity but also from their participation in social groups. By being in a group, a person gains a definition of who they are and what they stand for. The clinician can point out, therefore, that it is important after a transition that results in upheaval and uncertainty that the person should not withdraw and, to the extent possible, maintain their membership in such groups (Smeekes & Verkuyten, 2015).

Helping to manage regrets

Key literature-based findings

When taking a history during a clinical encounter, the person may express having significant regrets over something they did or did not do and describe feeling guilty, ashamed, or remorseful. The clinician can explain that it is quite common and in fact up to 90% of older adults experience one or more intense regrets (Landman, 1987; Wrosch, Bauer, & Scheier, 2005). The clinician can explain that regrets are especially likely to arise when people are older, given a greater need to look back and understand how a person has arrived where they are. In addition, when older a person is more likely to believe that there will be less opportunity going forward either to fulfill one's wishes or remedy errors that they feel they have made.

A clinician can point out that the presence of strong regrets has the potential to lower a person's well-being and unless challenged or "reframed" can cause the person to feel self-critical, contrite, and sad. Ruminating about regrets is especially likely to lower life satisfaction if the person regularly compares how they, or their circumstances, have turned out less well than the imagined, better alternative (Butler, 1963; Wrosch et al., 1995).

If a person describes being upset over what they did not do and wish they had done (i.e. acts of omission or "the road not taken"), the clinician can explain that this form of regret is more likely to cause them to remain distressed for longer periods of time compared to regrets over something that they actually did (i.e. acts of commission). While an act of commission may initially be more upsetting, over time, acts of omission are more enduring because a person is free to create almost any possible alternative to use to compare to what actually occurred . As a result, using this often idealized, wished-for alternative, the way the person's life has turned out is likely to viewed as less satisfying (Landman, 1987; Gilovich & Medvec, 1995).

Key strategies

If the person still has the ability and resources to fulfill a wish (e.g. travel and visit a friend not seen since childhood), or remedy an error that they feel they have made (e.g. apologize to a sibling for a disagreement after not talking to them for many years), the clinician can encourage them to take the action they are considering.

If the option is no longer available, or the person's declining personal resources do not allow the option of remedying the regret by action, which is often the case in late life, the clinician can point out that most people rely on internal strategies- they try to alter their perceptions and attitudes about their disappointments (Wrosch & Heckhausen, 2002). They consider the circumstances that existed at the time and try to understand why they did or did not do what they now regret (McQueen, 2017). During these discussions the clinician can empathize and encourage the person to be self-compassionate – to view themselves as simply human- imperfect and fallible; focus on the positive things that have occurred even though they made a choice that they now regret; and not over-idealize the outcomes attached to thoughts such as "what might have been is" or "if only I chose to" (Bauer, Wrosch, & Jobin, 2008).

Most importantly, the clinician can explain that when people can let go of their regrets and especially use their regrets as a life lesson, their well-being is relatively higher (Wrosch, Bauer, Miller, & Lupien, 2007). Thus, the clinician can offer to assist the person in considering what they can do now to "seize the day" and work to achieve new goals that might bring meaning and fulfillment in the present.

A frequently encountered challenge: Age-associated memory loss

Key literature based findings

A person is increasingly likely as they age to mention to a clinician that they are experiencing some degree of memory loss (Dixon, Rust, Feltmate, & See, 2007) and at times feel frustrated and embarrassed when they cannot perform everyday tasks in ways that they were able to in the past (Parikh, Troyer, Malone, & Murphy, 2015). They may also mention that they are afraid that their memory problems may worsen, have been avoiding learning opportunities anticipating that they will have difficulty and be frustrated, and are socializing less out of a fear that their memory problems will be "exposed" and they will then feel self-conscious (Frank & Kong,, 2008).

In fact not all aspects of memory decline with age. According to the memory systems perspective (Dixon et al., 2007), two memory systems most relevant to explaining the effects of aging on memory are the episodic memory system (i.e. a person's memory for personally experienced events or information) and the semantic memory system (i.e. a person's memory for acquiring and retaining generic facts, knowledge, and beliefs) (Hicks, Alexander, & Bahr, 2018).

There is an abundance of evidence that episodic memory declines as people get older in a relatively gradual fashion until people are in their mid-seventies and then more rapidly (Dixon et al., 2004; Dixon et al., 2007; Hicks et al., 2018). Unlike the decline in episodic memory, however, older adults are able to remember acquired and generic facts, knowledge, and beliefs as well as younger adults, although they may need more time to access and process this type of information (Backman & Nilsson, 1996).

Key strategies

A clinician can educate the person as to what typically changes in regard to memory with age – that about 40% of people aged 65 or older are likely to have specific memory impairments and occasionally forget specific events and experiences in their recent past as well as specific upcoming events and experiences (Koivisto et al., 1995); and as noted that most people notice a decline in the speed with which they process information (Koivisto et al., 1995).

The clinician can also point out that similar to most challenges associated with aging, a person's well-being is likely to be higher if the person feels that they are exerting as much personal control as they can and are preparing for occasions in which they may have a memory lapse (Gerstof et al., 2014). Specifically, a person in these circumstances can exert personal control by: learning, practicing, and executing memory compensatory strategies such as maintaining routines; employing external memory aids; and using personal associations when trying to retain new information (Simon, Yokomizo, & Bottino, 2012).

Old-old age

Key literature based findings

A person, for example, after being told during a visit that their chronic illness has progressed, may express the worry that they are entering into old-old age or late life. They might say that while they feel they can still compensate for many of the physical limitations that they have experienced and are still relatively independent, they notice that they are less able to overcome or rebound from obstacles and setbacks (Staudinger, Marsiske, & Baltes, 1995; Levy, 2009).

The clinician can explain that chronological age is a highly imprecise marker of old-old age and mention that there are two more helpful indicators. They are reserve capacity or the ability to be resilient, and subjective age – how old the person feels that they are, based on the cues that they receive from others and from the biomedical messages they get from their bodily systems (Karasik, Demissie, Cupples, & Kiel, 2005; Levy, 2009).

The clinician can point out that a person might tell if they have entered old-old age if they are less able to bounce back and compensate for any mental and physical limitations they are experiencing (Weiss, Sassenberg, & Freund, 2013). When they do enter old-old age, they are more likely to be aware of a significant decline in their sense of personal control and more conscious of the limited time that they have remaining to live, in part because of an increasing number of losses of family and friends (Johnson & Barer, 1993).

Key strategies

To maintain a person's well-being as they enter old-old age, face declining health and an increasing number of personal and social losses, a clinician can highlight the importance of engaging in pro-active planning. If the person is willing to engage in preventative and health-maintaining behavior and actively seek opportunities to experience pleasure and satisfaction, the clinician can point out that they are much more likely to experience a relatively high sense of well-being.

In addition, the clinician can explain that a person is more likely to maintain a sense of independence and mastery if they act as an autonomous agent in regard to the choices they have to make to the degree that they can, while simultaneously being as realistic about their decreasing ability to influence outcomes and their increasing need to depend on others.

The clinician can also mention that in keeping with Dylan Thomas's idea of not going "gentle into that good night", when a person is as active as they can be, they are more likely to experience a positive mood and pride that they still can be purposeful and productive (Herzog, Franks, Markus, & Holmberg, 1998; Rowe & Kahn, 1998). Lastly, the clinician can explain that while being active, they are especially likely to experience a positive mood and feel that life is worth living if they notice and savor occasions during which they feel appreciative and grateful (Wood, Froh, & Geraghty, 2010).

Loneliness, feelings of mattering, and a loss of purpose

Key literature findings

When talking to a person in late life, a clinician is likely to hear the person state that they feel lonely, do not matter sufficiently to others, and lack a purpose that "justifies" their continued existence. Compared to when they were younger, in old-old age people are likely to be socially isolated, have a smaller social network, and as a result, feel like an orphaned survivor (Carstensen, Isaacowitz, & Charles, 1999; Forster et al., 2018). Further, if their feelings of loneliness persist for a relatively long period of time, they are at increased risk of developing physical and mental health problems such as cognitive decline, a lack of energy, depression, and low self-esteem (Bouwman, Aartsen, van Tilburg, & Stevens, 2016).

The clinician can explain that people's social support systems do tend to shrink a great deal in very old age and that in fact there are likely to be fewer people who can pay attention to them and who they can rely on. The clinician can empathize with the likelihood that they might feel less noticed, useful, and valued, and even at times, feel that they do not have a convincing reason to continue to live (Froidevaux, Hirschi, & Wang, 2016).

The clinician can also point out that although these types of feelings are common, a person can still make a choice to be either apathetic, negative, and unwilling to exert effort to take care of their health or understand why they feel as they do, or they can be an active problem solver and see if there are ways that they might feel better (Boyle, Barnes, Buchman, & Bennett, 2009; Irving, Davis, & Collier, 2017).

Key strategies

If a person is motivated to be socially active and goal-oriented, the clinician can review the person's current social experiences and assess if they are being as active as they could be, accurately perceiving others' intentions and actions, and demonstrating social skill difficulties that may be adding to their feelings of social isolation.

The clinician can also question if the person is now being overly selective in who they choose to socialize with and can suggest that if they wish to feel they matter more, they need to spend time with people and be self-disclosing. The clinician can explain that people are more likely to feel connected to others and that they matter when they share their personal feelings and thoughts and while doing so, tell people what they wish to receive from them (Jourard, 1971).

Lastly, the clinician can point out that when someone feels lonely and without a purpose, joining a group is helpful, especially a group dedicated to a cause. By joining such a group, a person may feel part of a community and acquire a commitment to a set of goals.

Declining health and imminent death

Key literature-based findings

People in late life are likely to describe their life as very restricted and primarily organized around their medical difficulties. This is especially likely to be the case when a person has irreversible, progressive, and debilitating functional impairments as well as chronic diseases (Young, Frick, & Phelan, 2009). The clinician can inquire, and validate when accurate, that most people late in life have difficulty maintaining their sense of identity, experiencing positive emotions, and warding off negative emotions (Charmaz, 1983). In addition, they are likely to have difficulty "thinking forward" because while they know with certainty and feel anxious that their health will decline further, they are uncertain as to how and when these changes will occur. The clinician, in addition, can point out that many people at this stage of life feel a sense of grief for what they can no longer do – for the parts of themselves and their life that they have valued but can no longer experience (Smith, Borcheit, Maier, & Jopp, 2002).

If the person's health continues to decline and the person becomes aware that their death is imminent, they may be willing to acknowledge and share their feelings of terror with a clinician (Becker, 1973). The clinician can point out that typically people are better able to cope at this time if they review what they feel has been meaningful about their life, recognize what they have accomplished, and identify aspects of their life that they feel have had value (Sand, Olsson, & Strang, 2009). In addition, the clinician can highlight that people are better able to cope if they continue to select goals that they can look forward to (i.e. spending time with close friends, attending a grandchild's wedding). The clinician can explain that as a result of being able to anticipate and focus on an upcoming event, a person is likely to continue to feel they have a purpose and more likely to experience moments of satisfaction as they work to achieve a goal (Clayton, Butow, Arnold, & Tattersall, 2005).

Lastly, the clinician can mention still another way that people's actions can affect their well-being. They can resist the urge to withdraw, which frequently arises at this time. Instead, they can exert effort to maintain close connections with those they care about (Yalom, 2008) and be as active as they can (Chochinov, 2003).

Key strategies

A clinician can also offer to help a person identify a meaning framework that might bring them comfort and clarify what they have valued about their life. In addition, the clinician can encourage the person to maintain as many of their routines and activities as they can, and while doing so, be as much of an active decision-maker as possible (Rowe & Kahn, 1997). In this way, the clinician can explain, they are more likely to feel pride in being as autonomous as they can be as well as less anxious because, at least in some ways, they are being their "usual self" (Ouwehand, de Ridder, & Bensing, 2007).

As part of being their usual self, the clinician can point out that they have an opportunity to model how they wish to be remembered and, with this thought in mind, could use these aspired ways of acting as targets to strive for, as their energy and sense of personal control diminishes (Brandstädter, 1989). Lastly, the clinician can suggest that the person tell, and consider writing out, how and why the people they are close to matter to them (Chochinov, 2003).

Summing up

Based on the literature reviewed in this book, well-being is believed to be strongly affected by the degree of planning and effort people demonstrate in attempting to achieve and maintain the seven ingredients of well-being that have been described. In the face of the multiple, successive losses attached to aging – the loss of health, physical capacity and functionality, valued social relationships, and feelings of independence, efficacy, and usefulness, scholars who study aging have emphasized various factors they believe are especially important if people are to successfully cope with aging and experience a state of subjective well-being.

Some scholars, for example, believe that personal growth – the degree to which a person is engaged with life, maintains contact with other people, and participates in productive activities – is key (Rowe & Kahn, 1997). Other scholars believe that what is critical is being selective and optimizing activities and interests to facilitate resilience and maximize the chances of achieving desired goals; and when a person's capacities and resources dwindle, compensating by substituting alternative strategies or skills (Baltes & Baltes, 1990). Still other scholars propose that finding a personal meaning that endows life with significance, meaning, and fulfillment is critical (Wong, 1989).

The factors that seem to be especially important and exert a powerful effect on well-being as people age based on the perspectives presented in this book are the ability to take on an attitude of acceptance and the ability to exert personal control. As will be described, these factors can be considered two sides of one coin. By keeping these factors in mind, healthcare professionals can facilitate well-being during clinical encounters by helping people to both exert as much personal control as they can while recognizing occasions when a person needs to accept what they cannot change.

The essence of what is meant by acceptance is captured in the Serenity Prayer, attributed to the theologian-philosopher Reinhold Niebuhr (Shapiro, 2014). As stated, paraphrasing the words contained in the prayer, healthcare professionals can assist people in recognizing what they cannot change and in changing what they can. Particularly during times of uncertainty, loss, and dwindling health, when people are strongly challenged by what is beyond their control, a clinician can be an attachment figure who provides empathy and support and helps a person regulate the negative emotions that are likely to be present. During these conversations, the clinician can highlight that personal control is a prerequisite that needs to be exercised in order for the person to experience acceptance. It is only after a person has exerted effort, considered their choices, and attempted to do what they can to affect an outcome that they can know if they have to accept a less than desired result.

Finally, the clinician can highlight that acceptance is not a passive act or a synonym for resignation or submission. Rather, it is an active choice – a demonstration of agency. Especially in late life, when a person regularly confronts situations that cannot be affected through their direct actions, the clinician can explain that acceptance and personal control are entwined. The clinician can attempt to lessen the likelihood of the person experiencing despair by encouraging him or her to recognize that even though they cannot affect an external situation directly in the way that they wish, they can still make "internal" changes. They can alter their attitudes by flexibly adjusting their preferences and definitions of situations and by adopting viewpoints that facilitate social support, pride, and spiritual comfort. As a result of making such internal changes, a clinician can point out, a person is less likely to expend energy in the pursuit of unattainable goals and more likely to use their available resources to "seize the day" and live as fully and purposely as they can in the present.

References

Aartsen, M., & Jylha, M. (2011). Onset of loneliness in older adults: Results of a 28 year prospective study. *European Journal of Aging*, 8, 31–38.

Andersen-Ranberg, K., Schroll, M., & Jeune, B. (2001). Healthy centenarians do not exist, but autonomous centenarians do: A population-based study of morbidity. *Journal of the American Geriatric Society*, 49, 900–908.

Anderson, J.S. (2007). Pleasant, pleasurable, and positive activities. In L. L'Abate (Ed.), *Low-cost approaches to promote physical and mental health*. New York, NY: Springer.

Antonucci, T.C., Ajrouch, K.J., & Birditt, K.S. (2013). The convoy model: Explaining social relations from a multidisciplinary perspective. *The Gerontologist*, 54, 82–92.

Arbuckle, N.W., & de Vries, B. (1995). The long-term effects of later life spousal and parental bereavement on personal functioning. *The Gerontologist*, 35, 637–647.

Ardelt, M. (2004). Wisdom as an expert knowledge system: A critical review of a contemporary operationalization of an ancient concept. *Human Development*, 47, 304–307.

Aries, P. (1976). *Western attitudes toward death from the middle ages to the present*. Baltimore, MD: John Hopkins University Press.

Atchley, R.C. (1989). A continuity theory of normal aging. *The Gerontologist*, 29, 183–190.

Atchley, R.C. (1993). Continuity theory and the evolution of activity in later adulthood. In J. Kelly (Ed.), *Activity and aging* (pp. 5–16). Newbury Park, CA: Sage.

Atchley, R.C. (1997). Everyday mysticism: Spiritual development in later adulthood. *Journal of Adult Development*, 4, 123–134.

Baars, J. (2017a). Aging: Learning to live a finite life. *The Gerontologist*, 57, 969–976.

Baars, J. (2017b). Human aging, finite lives and the idealization of clocks. *Biogerontology*, 18, 285–292.

Backman, L., & Nilsson, L. (1996). Semantic memory functioning across the adult life span. *European Psychologist*, 1, 27–33.

Baltes, P.B. (1997). On the incomplete architecture of human ontogeny: Selection, optimization, and compensation as a foundation of developmental theory. *American Psychologist*, 52, 366–380.

Baltes, P.B. (1999). Lifespan psychology: Theory and application to intellectual functioning. *Annual Review of Psychology*, 50, 471–507.

Baltes, P.B., & Baltes, M.M. (1990). Psychological perspectives on successful aging: The model of selective optimization with compensation. In P.B. Baltes & M.M. Baltes

(Eds.), *Successful aging-perspectives from the behavioral sciences* (pp. 1–34). Cambridge: Cambridge University Press.

Baltes, M.M., & Carstensen, L.L. (1996). The process of successful aging. *Aging and Society*, 16, 397–422.

Baltes, P.B., & Smith, J. (1990). Toward a psychology of wisdom. In R.J. Sternberg (Ed.), *Wisdom: Its nature, origins, and development* (pp. 87–120). New York, NY: Cambridge University Press.

Baltes, P.B., & Staudinger, U.M. (2000). Wisdom: A metaheuristic (pragmatic) to orchestrate mind and virtue toward excellence. *American Psychologist*, 55, 122–126.

Bauer, I., & Wrosch, C. (2011). Making up for lost opportunities: The protective role of downward social comparisons for coping with regrets across adulthood. *Personality and Social Psychology Bulletin*, 37, 215–228.

Bauer, I., Wrosch, C., & Jobin, J. (2008). I'm better off than most other people: The role of social comparisons for coping with regret in young adulthood and old age. *Psychology and Aging*, 23, 800–811.

Baumeister, R.F. (1991). *Meanings of life*. New York, NY: Guilford Press.

Becker, E. (1973). *The denial of death*. New York, NY: The Free Press.

Bench, S.W., & Lench, H.C. (2013). On the function of boredom. *Behavioral Science*, 3, 459–472.

Bennett, K.M., & Soulsby, L.K. (2012). Wellbeing in bereavement and widowhood. *Illness, Crisis, & Loss*, 20, 321–337.

Benton, J.P., Christopher, A.N., & Walter, M.I. (2007). Death anxiety as a function of age. *Death Studies*, 31, 337–350.

Berlyne, D.E. (1971). *Aesthetics and psychobiology*. New York, NY: Appleton-Century-Croft.

Boston, P., Bruce, A., & Schreiber, R. (2011). Existential suffering in the palliative care setting: An integrated literature review. *Journal of Pain and Symptom Management*, 41, 604–618.

Bouwman, T.E., Aartsen, M.J., van Tilburg, T.G., & Stevens, N.L. (2016). Does stimulating various coping strategies alleviate loneliness? Results from an online friendship enrichment program. *Journal of Social and Personal Relations*, 34, 793–811.

Bowlby, J. (1960). Separation anxiety. *International Journal of Psycho-Analysis*, 41, 89–113.

Bowlby, J. (1980). *Attachment and loss I: Attachment*. New York, NY: Basic Books.

Bowlby, J. (1982). *A secure base*. New York, NY: Basic Books.

Boyle, P.A., Barnes, L.L., Buchman, A.S., & Bennett, D.A. (2009). Purpose in life is associated with mortality among community-dwelling older persons. *Psychosomatic Medicine*, 71, 574–579.

Brandstädter, J. (1989). Personal self-regulation of development: Cross-sequential analyses of development-related control beliefs and emotions. *Developmental Psychology*, 25, 96–108.

Brandstädter, J., & Greve, W. (1994). The aging self: Stabilizing and protective factors. *Developmental Review*, 14, 52–80.

Brandstädter, J., & Rothermund, K. (2002). The life course dynamics of goal pursuit and goal adjustment: A two process framework. *Developmental Review*, 22, 117–150.

Brier, N. (2015). *Enhancing self-control in adolescents*. New York, NY: Routledge.

Brown, K.W., & Ryan, R.M. (2003). The benefits of being present: Mindfulness and its role in psychological well-being. *Journal of Personality and Social Psychology*, 84, 822–848.

Burris, C.T., & Bailey, K. (2009). What lies ahead: Theory and measurement of after-death beliefs. *The International Journal for the Psychology of Religion*, 19, 173–186.

Butler, R.J. (1963). The life review: An interpretation of reminiscence in the aged. *Psychiatry*, 26, 65–76.

Butler, R.J. (2002). Life review. *Journal of Geriatric Psychiatry*, 35, 7–10.

Butrica, B.A., & Schaner, S.G. (2005). Satisfaction and engagement in retirement. *Perspectives on Productive Aging: The Urban Institute*, 2, July, 1–5.

Cacioppo, S., Grippo, A.J., London, S., Goosens, L., & Cacioppo, J.T. (2015). Loneliness: Clinical import and interventions. *Perspectives on Psychological Science*, 10, 238–249.

Carstensen, L.L. (1995). Evidence for a life-span theory of socio-emotional selectivity. *Current Directions in Psychological Science*, 4, 151–156.

Carstensen, L.L. (2006). The influence of a sense of time on human development. *Science*, 312, 1913–1915.

Carstensen, L.L., Isaacowitz, D.W., & Charles, S.T. (1999). Taking time seriously: A theory of socio-emotional selectivity. *American Psychologist*, 54, 165–181.

Carver, C.S., Scheier, M.F., & Weintraub, J.K. (1989). Assessing coping strategies: A theoretically based approach. *Journal of Personality and Social Psychology*, 56, 267–283.

Case, T.I., Fitness, J., Cairns, D.D., & Stevenson, R.J. (2004). Coping with uncertainty: Superstitious strategies and secondary control. *Journal of Applied Social Psychology*, 34, 848–871.

Cassell, E.J. (1976). *The healer's art*. Cambridge, MA: MIT Press.

Chappell, N.I., & Badger, M. (1989). Social isolation and well-being. *Journal of Gerontology*, 44, 169–176.

Charles, S., & Carstensen, L.L. (2010). Social and emotional aging. *Annual Review of Psychology*, 61, 383–409.

Charmaz, K. (1983). Loss of self: A fundamental form of suffering in the chronically ill. *Sociology of Health and Illness*, 5, 168–195.

Chipperfield, J.G., Newall, N.E., Perry, R.P., Stewart, T.L., Bailis, D.S., & Ruthig, J.C. (2012). Sense of control in late life: Health and survival implications. *Personality and Social Psychology Bulletin*, 38, 1081–1092.

Chochinov, H.M. (2003). Thinking outside the box: Depression, hope, and meaning at the end of life. *Journal of Palliative Medicine*, 6, 973–977.

Chochinov, H.M., Hack, T., McClement, S., Kristjanson, L.K., & Harlos, M. (2002). Dignity in the terminally ill: A developing empirical model. *Social Science & Medicine*, 54, 433–443.

Choron, J. (1974). *Death and modern man*. New York, NY: Macmillan.

Clayton, J.M., Butow, P.N., Arnold, R.M., & Tattersall, M.H. (2005). Fostering coping and nurturing hope when discussing the future with terminally ill cancer patients and their caregivers. *Cancer*, 103, 1965–1975.

Connidis, I.A., & Davies, L. (1990). Confidants and companions in later life: The place of family and friends. *Journal of Gerontology*, 45, S141–149.

Crowther, M.A., Parker, M.W., Achenbaum, W.A., Larimore, W.L., & Koenig, H.G. (2002). Rowe and Kahn's model of successful aging revisited: Positive spirituality-the forgotten factor. *The Gerontologist*, 42, 61–620.

Csikszentmihalyi, M. (1975). *Beyond boredom and anxiety*. San Francisco, CA: Jossey-Bass.

Csikszentmihalyi, M. (1996). *Creativity: Flow and the psychology of discovery and invention*. New York, NY: HarperCollins.

Cummins, R.A., & Wooden, M. (2013). Personal resilience in times of crises: The implications of SWB homeostasis and set points. *Journal of Happiness Studies*, doi:10.1007/s10902–10013–9481–9484.

Davies E., & Cartwright, S. (2011). Psychological and psychosocial predictors of attitudes to working past normal retirement age. *Employee Relations*, 33, 249–268.

de Jong Gierveld, J., & Havens, B. (2004). Cross-national comparison of social isolation and loneliness: Introduction and overview. *Canadian Journal on Aging*, 23, 109–123.

d'Epinay, C.J., Cavalli, S., & Spini, D. (2003). The death of a loved one: Impact on health and relationships in very old age. *Omega*, 47, 265–284.

d'Epinay, C.J., Cavalli, S., & Guillet, L.A. (2009–2010). Bereavement in very old age: Impact on health and relationships of the loss of a spouse, a child, a sibling, or a close friend. *Omega*, 60, 301–325.

D'Esposito, M.D., & Gazzaley, A. (2011). Can age-associated memory decline be treated? *The New England Journal of Medicine*, 365, 1346–1347.

de Vries, B., & Johnson, C. (2002). The death of friends in later life. *Advances in Life Course Research*, 7, 299–324.

Diener, E. (1984). Subjective well-being. *Psychological Bulletin*, 95, 542–575.

Diener, E., & Ryan, K. (2009). Subjective well-being: A general overview. *South African Journal of Psychology*, 39, 391–406.

Diener, E., Suh, E.M., Lucas, R.E., & Smith, H.L. (1999). Subjective well-being: Three decades of progress. *Psychological Bulletin*, 125, 276–302.

Dietz, B.E. (1996). The relationship of aging to self-esteem: The relative effects of maturation and role accumulation. *International Journal of Aging*, 43, 249–266.

Dingemans, E. (2012). Bridge employment after early retirement: A bridge to better post-retirement well-being of older adults? Netspar Theses. Retrieved from https://netspar.nl/en/publication/bridge-employment-after-early-retirement-a-bridge-to-better-postretirement-well-being-of-older-adults/.

Dingemans, E., & Henkens, K. (2015). How do retirement dynamics influence mental well-being in later life? A 10 year panel study. *Scandinavian Journal of Work Environment Health*, 41, 16–23.

Dixon, A.L. (2007). Mattering in the later years: Older adults' experience of mattering to others, purpose in life, depression, and wellness. *Adultspan*, 6, 83–95.

Dixon, R.A., Rust, R.B., Feltmate, S.E., & See, S.K. (2007). Memory and aging: Selected research directions and application issues. *Canadian Psychology*, 48, 67–76.

Dixon, R.A., Wahlin, A., Maitland, S.B., Hultsch, D.F., Hertzog, C., & Backman, L. (2004). Episodic memory change in late adulthood: Generalizability across samples and performance indices. *Memory and Cognition*, 32, 768–778.

Dogan, T., Totan, T., & Sapmaz, F. (2013). The role of self-esteem, psychological well-being, emotional self-efficacy, and affect balance on happiness: A path model. *European Scientific Journal*, 9, 31–42.

Dunkel, C.S., & Worsley, S.K. (2016). Does identity continuity promote personality stability? *Journal of Research in Personality*, 65, 11–15.

Dykstra, P.A., & de Jong Gierveld, J. (2004). Gender and marital history differences in emotional and social loneliness among Dutch older adults. *Canadian Journal on Aging*, 23, 141–155.

Eastwood, J.D., Frischen, A., Fenske, M.J., & Smilek, D. (2012). The unengaged mind: Defining boredom in terms of attention. *Perspectives in Psychological Science*, 7, 482–495.

Edward, J. (2016). Friends in old age. *Clinical Social Work*, 44, 198–203.

Ekerdt, D.J., & DeViney, S. (1990). On defining persons as retired. *Journal of Aging Studies*, 4, 211–229.

Elliot, G.C., Kao, S., & Grant, A. (2004). Mattering: Empirical validation of a social-psychological concept. *Self and Identity*, 3, 339–354.

Ellwardt, T., van Tilburg, T., Aartsen, M., Wittek, R., & Steverink, N. (2015). Personal networks and mortality risk in older adults: A twenty year longitudinal study. *PLOS One*, March 3, 2015.

Elpidorou, A. (2014). The bright side of boredom. *Frontiers in Psychology*, 5, 1245.

Erikson, E.H. (1963). *Childhood and society*, Second Edition. New York, NY: W.W. Norton & Company.

Erikson, E.H. (1985). *The life cycle completed: A review*. New York, NY: W.W. Norton & Company.

Erikson, E., Erikson, J.M., & Kivnik, H.Q. (1986). *Vital involvement in old age*. New York, NY: W. W. Norton & Company.

Fazio, E.M. (2010). Sense of mattering in late life. In W.R. Avison, C.S., Aneshemi, S., Schieman, & B. Wheaton (Eds.), *Advances in the conceptualization of the stress process* (pp. 149–167). New York, NY: Springer.

Feeney, B.C., & Collins, N.L. (2015). A new look at social support: A theoretical perspective on thriving through relationships. *Personality and Social Psychology Review*, 19, 113–147.

Feldman, D.C. (1994). The decision to retire early: A review and conceptualization. *Academy of Management Review*, 19, 285–311.

Flynn, C.P., & Kunkel, S.R. (1987). Deprivation, compensation, and conceptions of an afterlife. *Sociological Analysis*, 48, 58–72.

Folkman, S., & Greer, S. (2000). Promoting psychological well-being in the face of serious illness: when theory, research and practice inform each other. *PsychoOncology*, 9, 11–19.

Forster, F., Stein, J., Löbner, M., Pabst, A., Angermeyer, M.C., König, H.H., & Riedel-Heller, S.G. (2018). Loss experiences in old age and their impact on the social network and depression- results of the Leipzig Longitudinal Study of the Aged (LEILA 75+). *Journal of Affective Disorders*, 241, 94–102.

Frank, M.J., & Kong, L. (2008). Learning to avoid in older age. *Psychology and Aging*, 23, 392–398.

Frank, L., Lloyd, A., Flynn, J.A., Kleinman, L., Matza, L.S., Margolis, M.K., … Bullock, R. (2006). Impact of cognitive impairment on mild dementia patients and their informants. *International Psychogeriatrics*, 18, 151–162.

Frankl, V. (1984). *Man's search for meaning: An introduction to logotherapy*. New York, NY: Simon & Schuster.

Fredrickson, B., & Carstensen, L.L. (1990). Choosing social partners: How old age and anticipated endings make people more selective. *Psychology and Aging*, 5, 163–171.

Froidevaux, A., Hirschi, A., & Wang, M. (2016). The role of mattering as an overlooked key challenge in retirement planning and adjustment. *Journal of Vocational Behavior*, 94, 57–69.

Fry, P.M., & Debats, D.L. (2002). Self-efficacy beliefs as predictors of loneliness and psychological distress in older adults. *International Journal of Aging and Human Development*, 55, 233–269.

Gana, K., Alaphillippe, D., & Bailly, N. (2004). Positive illusions and mental and physical health in later life. *Aging & Mental Health*, 8, 58–64.

Gerstorf, D., Ram, N., Schupp, J., Heckhausen, J., Infurna, F.J. & Wagner, G. (2014). Perceived personal control buffers terminal decline in well-being. *Psychology and Aging*, 29, 612–625.

Gilleard, C., & Higgs, P. (2010). Frailty, disability, and old age: A reappraisal. *Health*, 15, 475–490.

Gesser, G., Wong, P., & Reker, G. (1987–1988). Death attitudes across the life span: The development and validation of the death attitude profile (DAP). *Omega: The Journal of Death and Dying*, 18, 113–128.

Gilovich, T., & Medvec, V.H. (1995). The experience of regret: What, when, and why? *Psychological Review*, 102, 379–395.

Gollwitzer, P.M. (1999). Implementation intentions: Strong effects of simple plans. *American Psychologist*, 54, 493–503.

Greenberg, J., Solomon, S., & Pyszcynski, T. (1997). Terror Management Theory of self-esteem and cultural world views: Empirical evidence and conceptual refinements. *Advances in Experimental Social Psychology*, 29, 61–139.

Gregory, T., Nettlebeck, T., & Wilson, C. (2010). Openness to experience and successful aging. *Personality and Individual Differences*, 48, 895–899.

Gupta, R., & Hershey, D.A. (2016). Cross-national differences in goals for retirement: The case of India and the United States. *Journal of Cross Cultural Gerontology*, 31, 221–236.

Hansen, T., Aartsen, M., Slagsvold, B., & Deindl, C. (2018). Dynamics of volunteering and life satisfaction in midlife and old age: Findings from 12 European countries. *Social Sciences*, May 4, 2018.

Hartog, J. (1980). The anlage and ontology of loneliness. In J. Hartog, J.R. Audy, & Y.A. Cohen (Eds.), *The Anatomy of Loneliness*. New York, NY: International University Press.

Hershey, D.A., Jacobs-Lawson, J.M., & Neukam, K.N. (2002). Influence of age and gender on workers goals for retirement. *International Journal of Aging and Human Development*, 55, 163–179.

Herzog, A.R., Franks, M.M., Markus, H.R., & Holmberg, D. (1998). Activities and well-being in older age: Effects of self-concept and educational attainment. *Psychology and Aging*, 13, 179–185.

Hicks, R.E., Alexander, V.E., & Bahr, M. (2018). Explicit and implicit memory loss in aging. *International Journal of Psychological Studies*, 10, 40–52.

Hidi, S., & Renninger, K.A. (2006). The four-phase model of interest development. *Educational Psychologist*, 41, 111–127.

Hill, R.D. (2011). A positive aging perspective for guiding geropsychology interventions. *Behavior Therapy*, 42, 66–77.

Hoelter, J.W. (1979). Multidimensional treatment of fear of death. *Journal of Consulting and Clinical Psychology*, 47, 996–999.

Holahan, C.K., & Suzuki, R. (2006). Motivational factors in health promoting behavior in later aging. *ACT Adaptation Aging*, 30, 47–60.

Holahan, C.K., Holahan, C.J., Velasquez, K.E., & North, R.J. (2008). Family support, family income and happiness: A 10-year perspective. *International Journal of Aging and Human Development*, 66, 229–241.

Huta, V., & Ryan (2010). Pursuing pleasure in virtue: Differential and overlapping well-being benefits of hedonic and eudaimonic motives. *Journal of Happiness Studies*, 11, 735–762.

Irving, J., Davis, S., & Collier, A. (2017). Aging with purpose: Systematic search and review of literature pertaining to older adults and purpose. *The International Journal of Aging and Human Development*, 85, 403–437.

Isaacowitz, D.M., & Smith, J. (2003). Positive and negative affect in very old age. *Journal of Gerontology*, 58b, 143–152.

Jeste, D.V., & Oswald, A.J. (2014). Individual and societal wisdom: Explaining the paradox of human aging and well-being. *Psychiatry*, 77, 317–330.

Jeste, D.V., Savla, G.H., Thompson, W.K., Vahia, I.V., Glorioso, D.K., Martin, A. S., … Depp, C.A. (2013). Older age is associated with more successful aging: Role of resilience and depression. *American Journal of Psychiatry*, 170, 188–196.

Johnson, C.L., & Barer, B.M. (1993). Coping and a sense of control among the oldest: An exploratory analysis. *Journal of Aging Studies*, 7, 67–80.

Joosten-Weyn Banningh, L.W.A., Kessels, R.P.C., Olde Rikert, M.G.M., Geleijns-Lanting, C.E., & Kraaimaat, F.W. (2008). A cognitive behavioral group therapy for patients with mild cognitive impairment and their significant others: Feasibility and preliminary results. *Clinical Rehabilitation*, 22, 731–740.

Jourard, S.M. (1971). *The transparent self*. New York, NY: Van Nostrand Reinhold.

Kahn, R.L., & Antonucci, T.C. (1980). Convoys over the life course: Attachment, roles and social support. In P.B. Baltes & O.J. Brim (Eds.), *Life-span development and behavior* (pp. 254–283). San Diego, CA: Academic Press.

Karasik, D., Demissie, S., Cupples, & Kiel, D.P. (2005). Disentangling the genetic determinants of human aging: Biological age as an alternative to the use of survival measures. *Journal of Gerontology*, 60a, 574–587.

Kasden, T. (2009). *Curious?*New York, NY: Harper.

Kashdan, T.B., Rose, P., & Fincham, F.D. (2004). Curiosity and exploration: Facilitating positive subjective experiences and personal growth opportunities. *Journal of Personality Assessment*, 82, 291–305.

Kastenbaum, R.J. (2009). *Death, society, and human experience*. Boston, MA: Allyn & Bacon.

Kim, E.S., Strecher, V.J., & Ryff, C.D. (2014). Purpose in life and use of preventive health care services. *Proceedings of the National Academy of Sciences*, 111, 16331–16336.

Kim, J.E., & Moen, P. (2002). Retirement transitions, gender, and psychological well-being: A life course, ecological model. *Journal of Gerontology, Psychological Sciences*, 57b, 212–222.

Kirkegaard, S. (1957). *The concept of dread*. Princeton, NJ: University Press.

Klass, D., Silverman, P., & Nickman, S. (Eds.) (1996). *Continuing bonds: New understandings of grief*. Philadelphia, PA: Taylor & Francis.

Klug, L., & Sinha, A. (1987). Death acceptance: A two component formulation and scale. *Omega: Journal of Death and Dying*, 18, 229–235.

Koivisto, K., Reinikainen, K., Hänninen, T., Vanhanen, M., Helkala, E.L., Mykkänen, L., … Riekkinen, P.J., Snr (1995). Prevalence of age-associated memory impairment in a randomly selected population from eastern Finland. *Neurology*, 45, 741–747.

Krause, N., & Shaw, B.E. (2003). Role-specific control, personal meaning, and health in late life. *Research on Aging*, 25, 559–586.

Landman, J. (1987). Regret: A theoretical and conceptual analysis. *Journal for the theory of Social Behavior*, 17, 135–160.

Lang, F.R., & Carstensen, L.F. (1994). Close emotional relationships in late life: Further support for proactive aging in the social domain. *Psychology and Aging*, 9, 315–324.

Lang, F.R., & Carstensen, L.L. (2002). Time counts: Future time perspective, goals, and social relationships. *Psychology and Aging*, 17, 125–139.

Lennings, C.J. (2000). Optimism, Satisfaction and time perspective in the elderly. *International Journal of Aging and Human Development*, 51, 167–181.

Leong, F.T., & Schneller, G.R. (1993). Boredom proneness: Temperamental and cognitive components. *Personality and Individual Differences*, 14, 233–239.

Levy, B. (2009). Stereotype embodiment: A psychosocial approach to aging. *Current Directions in Psychological Science*, 18, 332–336.

Lifton, R. (1973). The sense of immortality: On death and the continuity of life. *The American Journal of Psychoanalysis*, 33, 3–15.

Lifton, R. (1976). *The life of the self: Toward a new psychology*. New York, NY: Simon & Schuster.

Lifton, J., & Olson, E. (1974). *Living and dying*. New York, NY: Praeger.

Lodi-Smith, J., Spain, S.M., Cologgi, K., & Roberts, B.W. (2017). Development of identity clarity and content in adulthood. *Journal of Personality and Social Psychology*, 112, 755–768.

Lopata, H.Z. (1996). *Current widowhood: Myths and realities*. London: Sage.

Luong, G., Charles, S.T., & Fingerman, K.L. (2011). Better with age: Social relationships across adulthood. *Journal of Social and Personality Relations*, 28, 9–23.

Lyubomirsky, S. (2008). *The how of happiness: A scientific approach to getting the life you want*. New York, NY: Penguin Press.

Mak, L., & Marshall, S.K. (2004). Perceived mattering in young adults' romantic relationships. *Journal of Social and Personal Relationships*, 21, 469–486.

Marks, N.F., Jun, H., & Song, J. (2007). Death of parents and adult psychological and physical well-being. *Journal of Family Issues*, 28, 1611–1638.

Markus, H., & Nurius, P. (1986). Possible selves. *American Psychologist*, 41, 954–969.

Marshall, S.K. (2001). Do I matter? Construct validation of adolescents' perceived mattering to parents and friends. *Journal of Adolescence*, 24, 473–490.

Martin, P., Kliegel, M., Rott, C., Poon, L.W., & Johnson, M.A. (2008). Age differences and changes in coping behavior in three age groups: Findings from the Georgia Centenerian Study. *International Journal of Aging*, 66, 97–114.

Maslow, A. (1971). *The farther reaches of human nature*. New York, NY: The Viking Press.

McCrae, R.R. (1992). Openness to experience as a basic dimension of personality. Paper presented at the Annual Convention of the American Psychological Association. Washington, DC, August 14–18.

McKnight, P.E., & Kashdan, T.B. (2009). Purpose in life as a system that creates and sustains health and well-being: An integrative, testable theory. *Review of General Psychology*, 13, 242–251.

McQueen, P. (2017). When should we regret? *International Journal of Philosophical Studies*, 25, 608–623.

Mendoza-Nunez, V.M. (2016). What is the onset age of human aging and old age? *International Journal of Gerontology*, 10, 56.

Menninger, W. (1999). Adaptional challenges and coping in late life. *Bulletin of the Menninger Clinic*, 63, a4–a15.

Miller, L.M.S., & Lachman, M.E. (1999). The sense of control and cognitive aging: Toward a model of mediational processes. In Hess, T.M. & Blanchard-Fields, F. (Eds.) *Social cognition and aging*. New York, NY: Academic Press (pp. 17–41).

Molton, I.V., & Jensen, M.P. (2010). Aging and disability: Biopsychosocial perspectives. *Physical Medicine and Rehabilitation Clinics of North America*, 21, 253–265.

Montross, L.P., Depp, C., Reichstadt, J., Golshan, S., Moore, D., Sitzer, D., & Jesie, D. V. (2006). Correlates of self-rated successful aging among community-dwelling older adults. *American Journal of Geriatric Psychiatry*, 14, 43–51.

Moss, M.S., Lesher, E.L., & Moss, S.Z. (1986–1987). Impact of the death of an adult child on elderly parents: Some observations. *Omega*, 17, 209–218.

Moss, S.Z., & Moss, M.M. (1989). The impact of the death of an elderly sibling. *The American Behavioral Scientist*, 33, 94–106.

Neff, K.A. (2003). Self-compassion: An alternative conceptualization of a healthy attitude toward oneself. *Self and Identity*, 2, 85–102.

Neimeyer, R.A. (2000). Searching for the meaning of meaning: Grief therapy and the process of reconstruction. *Death Studies*, 24, 541–558.

Neimeyer, R.A., Wittkowski, J., & Moser, R.P. (2003). Psychological research on death attitudes: An overview and evaluation. *Death Studies*, 28, 309–340.

Nekolaichuk, C.L., & Bruera, E. (1998). On the nature of hope in palliative care. *Journal of Palliative Care*, 14, 36–41.

Olds, T., Burton, N.W., Sprod, J., Maher, C., Ferrar, K., Brown, W.J., … Dumuid, D. (2018). One day you'll wake up and won't have to go to work: The impact of changes in time use on mental health following retirement. *PloS ONE*, 13, e0199605.

Osborne, J.W. (2012). Psychological effects of the transition to retirement. *Canadian Journal of Counseling and Psychotherapy*, 46, 45–58.

Ouwehand, C., de Ridder, D.T., & Bensing, J.M. (2007). A review of successful aging models: Proposing proactive coping as an important additional strategy. *Clinical Psychology Review*, 27, 873–884.

Palgi, Y., & Shmotkin, D. (2010). The predicament of time near the end of life: Time perspective trajectories of life satisfaction among the old-old. *Aging & Mental Health*, 14, 577–586.

Palys, T.S., & Little, B.R. (1983). Perceived life satisfaction and the organization of personal project systems. *Journal of Personality and Social Psychology*, 44, 1221–1230.

Panksepp, J. (1998). *Affective neuroscience: The foundations of human and animal emotion*. New York, NY: Oxford University Press.

Paradise, A.W., & Kernis, M.H. (2002). Self-esteem and psychological well-being: Implications of fragile self-esteem. *Journal of Social and Clinical Psychology*, 21, 345–361.

Parikh, P., Troyer, A.K., Malone, A.A., & Murphy, K.J. (2015). The impact of memory changes on daily life in normal aging and mild cognitive impairment. *The Gerontologist*, 56, 877–885.

Park, H.L., O'Connell, J.E., & Thompson, R.G. (2003). A systematic review of cognitive decline in the generally elderly population. *International Journal of Geriatric Psychiatry*, 18, 1121–1134.

Pennebaker, J.W. (1997). Writing about emotional experiences as a therapeutic process. *Psychological Science*, 8, 162–166.

Pinquart, M. (2002). Creating and maintaining purpose in life in old age: A meta-analysis. *Ageing International*, 27, 90–114.

Pyszcznski, T., Wicklund, R., Floresku, S., Gauch, G., Solomon, S., & Greenberg, J. (1996). Whistling in the dark: Exaggerated consensus estimates in response to incremental reminders of mortality. *Psychological Science*, 7, 333–336.

Qualter, P., Vanhalst, J., Harris, R., Van Roekel, E., Lodder, G., Bangee, M., ... Verhagen, M. (2015). Loneliness across the life span. *Perspectives on Psychological Science*, 10, 250–264.

Reker, G.T., Peacock, E.J., & Wong, P. (1987). Meaning and purpose in life and well-being: A life span perspective. *Journal of Gerontology*, 42, 44–49.

Roberto, K.A., & Stanis, P.I. (1994). Reactions of older women to the death of close friends. *Omega*, 29, 17–27.

Robins, R.W., & Trzesniewski, K.H. (2005). Self esteem development across the life span. *Current Directions in Psychological Science*, 14, 158–162.

Rodriquez-Diaz, M.T., Perez-Marfil, M.N., & Cruz-Quintana, F. (2016). Coexisting with dependence and well-being: The results of a pilot study intervention on 75–99 year-old individuals. *International Geriatrics*, 28, 2067–2078.

Rokach, A. (2014). Addressing loneliness in old age. *International Journal of Psychology Research*, 9, 317–332.

Rook, K.S. (1984). Promoting social bonding: Strategies for helping the lonely and socially isolated. *American Psychologist*, 39, 1389–1407.

Rook, K.S. (2009). Gaps in social support resources in later life: An adaptional challenge in need of further research. *Journal of Social and Personality Relationships*, 26, 103–112.

Rook, K.S., & Charles, S.T. (2017). Close social ties and health in later life: Strength and vulnerabilities. *American Psychologist*, 72, 567–577.

Rostila, M., & Saarela, J.M. (2011). Time does not heal all wounds: Mortality following the death of a parent. *Journal of Marriage and Family*, 73, 236–249.

Rothbaum, R., Weisz, J.R., & Snyder, S.S. (1982). Changing the world and changing the self: A two process model of perceived control. *Journal of Personality and Social Psychology*, 42, 5–37.

Rothermund, K., & Brandstädter, J. (2003). Coping with deficits and losses in later life: From compensatory action to accomodation. *Psychology and Aging*, 18, 896–905.

Rowe, J.W., & Kahn, R.L. (1997). Successful aging. *The Gerontologist*, 37, 433–440.

Rowe, J.W., & Kahn, R.L. (1998). *Successful aging*. New York, NY: Pantheon.

Ryan, R., & Deci, E.L. (2001). On happiness and human potentials: A review of research on hedonic and eudaimonic well-being. *Annual Review of Psychology*, 52, 141–166.

Ryff, C.D. (1989). Happiness is everything, or is it? Explorations in the meaning of psychological well-being. *Journal of Personality and Social Psychology*, 57, 1069–1081.

Ryff, C.D. (1995). Psychological well-being in adult life. *Current Directions in Psychological Science*, 6, 286–295.

Ryff, C.D., & Keyes, C.L. (1995). The structure of psychological well-being revisited. *Journal of Personality and Social Psychology*, 69, 719–727.

Saklofske, D.H., & Yackulic, R. (1989). Personality predictors of loneliness. *Personality and Individual Differences*, 10, 467–472.

Salthouse, T.A. (2006). Mental exercise and mental aging: Evaluating the validity of the use it or lose it hypothesis. *Perspectives on Psychological Science*, 1, 68–87.

Sand, L., Olsson, M., & Strang, O. (2009). Coping strategies in the presence of one's own death. *Journal of Pain and Symptom Management*, 37, 13–22.
Schafer, M.H., & Shipee, T.P. (2010). Age identity in context: Stress and the subjective side of aging. *Social Psychology Quarterly*, 73, 245–264.
Schulz, R., & Heckhausen, J. (1999). A life span model of successful aging. *American Psychologist*, 51, 702–714.
Seligman, M.E. (2002). *Authentic happiness: Using positive psychology for lasting fulfillment.* New York, NY: Free Press.
Seligman, M.E. (2011). *Flourish*. New York, NY: Simon & Schuster.
Seligman, M.E., Steen, T.A., Park, N., & Peterson, C. (2005). Positive psychology progress: Empirical validation of interventions. *American Psychologist*, 5, 410–421.
Sewdas, R., de Wind, A., van der Zwaan, L., & van der Borg, W.E. (2017). Why older workers work beyond the retirement age: A qualitative study. *BMC Public Health*, 17, 672.
Shapiro, F.R. (April 28, 2014). Who wrote the Serenity Prayer? *The Chronicle of Higher Education*, Washington, DC.
Simon, S.S., Yokomizo, J.E., & Bottino, C.N. (2012). Cognitive intervention in amnestic Mild Cognitive Impairment: A systematic review. *Neuroscience Biobehavioral Review*, 36, 1163–1178.
Skinner, E.A. (1996). A guide to constructs of control. *Journal of Personality and Social Psychology*, 71, 549–570.
Sklar, F., & Hartley, S.F. (1990). Close friends as survivors: Bereavement patterns in a "hidden" population. *Omega: Journal of Death and Dying*, 21, 103–112.
Smeekes, A., & Verkuyten, M. (2015). The presence of the past: Identity continuity and group dynamics. *European Review of Social Psychology*, 26, 162–202.
Smith, J., Borcheit, M., Maier, H., & Jopp, D. (2002). Health and well-being in the young old and oldest old. *Journal of Social Issues*, 58, 715–732.
Smith, J.L., Wagaman, J., & Handley, I.M. (2009). Keeping it dull or making it fun: Task variation as a function of promotion verses prevention focus. *Motivation and Emotion*, 33, 150–160.
Sneed, J.R., & Whitbourne, S.K. (2003). Identity processes and self-consciousness in middle and later adulthood. *The Journals of Gerontology – Series B: Psychological Sciences and Social Sciences*, 58, 375–388.
Solano, C.H., Batten, P.G., & Parish, E.A. (1982). Loneliness and patterns of self-disclosure. *Journal of Personality and Social Psychology*, 43, 524–531.
Spahni, S., Bennett, K.M., & Perrig-Chiello, P. (2015). Psychological adaptation to spousal bereavement in old age. The role of trait resilience, marital history, and context of death. *Gerontology*, 61, 456–468.
Staudinger, U.M., Marsiske, M., & Baltes, P.B. (1995). Resilience and reserve capacity in later adulthood: Potentials and limits across the life span. In D. Cicchetti & D.J. Cohen (Eds.), *Developmental psychopathology* (Vol. 2: Risk, Disorder, and Adaption; pp. 801–847). New York, NY: Wiley.
Stephan, Y. (2009). Openness to experience and active older adults' life satisfaction: A trait and facet-level analysis. *Personality and Individual Differences*, 47, 637–641.
Stephan, Y., Sutin, A.R., & Terracciano, A. (2015). How old do you feel? The role of age discrimination and biological aging in subjective age. *PLOS One*, 10(3), March 4.
Steptoe, A., & Fancourt, D. (2019). Leading a meaningful life at older ages and its relationship with social engagement, prosperity, health, biology, and time use. *PNAS*, 116, 1207–1212.

Strain, L.A., & Chappell, N.L. (1982). Confidants. *Research on Aging*, 4, 479–502.

Syverson, C. (2011). What determines productivity? *Journal of Economic Literature*, 49, 326–365.

Tang, F., Choi, E., & Goode, R. (2013). Older Americans employment and retirement. *Ageing International*, 38, 82–94.

Taylor, S.E. (1983). Adjustment to threatening events: A theory of cognitive adaption. *American Psychologist*, 38, 1161–1173.

Tiilikainen, E., & Seppanen, M. (2017). Lost and unfulfilled relationships behind emotional loneliness in old age. *Ageing & Society*, 37, 1068–1088.

Timmer, E., Westerhof, G., & Dittman-Kohli, F. (2005). "When looking back on my past life I regret…": Retrospective regret in the second half of life. *Death Studies*, 29, 625–644.

Tinker, A. (1993). When does old age start? *International Journal of Geriatric Psychiatry*, 8, 711–716.

Tomer, A., & Eliason, G. (2001). Towards a comprehensive model of death anxiety. *Death Studies*, 20, 343–365.

Torges, C.M., Stewart, A.J., & Nolen-Hoeksema, S. (2008). Regret resolution, aging, and adapting to loss. *Psychology and Aging*, 23, 169–180.

Tornstam, L. (1989). Gero-transcendence: A reformulation of the disengagement theory. *Aging*, 1, 55–63.

Troyer, A.K., Murphy, K.J., Anderson, N.D., Moscovitch, M., & Craik, F.I. (2008). Changing everyday memory behavior in amnestic mild cognitive impairments: A randomized controlled trial. *Neuropsychological Rehabilitation*, 28, 65–88.

Trumble, W.R. (2002). *Shorter Oxford University dictionary*, Fifth Edition. New York, NY: Oxford University Press.

United Nations (2015). World population ageing 2015. New York, NY: Department of Economic and Social Affairs. Population Division (ST/ASA/SER.A390). Retrieved from https://www.un.org/en/development/desa/population/publications/pdf/ageing/WPA2015_Report.pdf.

van den Bos, K. (2009). Making sense of life: The existential self trying to deal with personal uncertainty. *Psychological Inquiry*, 20, 197–217.

Van Tilburg, W.A., & Igou, E.R. (2012). On boredom: Lack of challenge and meaning as distinct boredom experiences. *Motivation and Emotion*, 36, 181–194.

van Wijngaarden, E., Leget, C., & Goossensen, A. (2015). Ready to give up on life: The lived experience of elderly people who feel life is completed and no longer worth living. *Social Science & Medicine*, 138, 257–264.

Verhaeghen, P., Geraerts, N., & Marcoen, A. (2000). Memory complaints, coping, and well-being in old age: A systemic approach. *The Gerontologist*, 40, 540–548.

Victor, C.R., Scambler, S.J., Bowling, A., & Bond, J. (2005). The prevalence of, and risk for, loneliness in later life: A survey of older people in Great Britain. *Ageing and Society*, 25, 357–375.

Voldanovich, S.J., & Watt, J.D. (1999). The relationship between time structure and boredom proneness: An investigation within two cultures. *The Journal of Social Psychology*, 139, 143–152.

Wang, M., Henkens, K., & van Solinge, H. (2011). Retirement adjustment: A review of theoretical and empirical advancements. *American Psychologist*, 66, 204–213.

Wang, Y., & Perez-Quinones, M.A. (2014). Exploring the role of prospective memory in location-based reminders. September 13–17, UBICOMP'14 Adjunct, Seattle, WA.

Ward, R., LaGory, M., & Sherman, S. (1982). The relative importance of social ties. Paper presented at the Annual Scientific Meeting of the Gerontological Society (35th, Boston, MA), November, 19–23.

Watkins, P.C., Woodward, K., Stone, T., & Kolts, R.L. (2003). Gratitude and happiness: Development of a measure of gratitude, and relations with subjective well-being. *Social Behavior and Personality: An International Journal*, 31, 431–451.

Weinstein, L., Xie, X., & Cleanthous, C.C. (1995). Purpose in life, boredom, and volunteerism in a group of retirees. *Psychological Reports*, 76, 482.

Weiss, D., Sassenberg, K., & Freund, A.M. (2013). When feeling different pays off: How older adults can counteract negative age-related information. *Psychology and Aging*, 28, 1140–1146.

Weiss, R.S. (Ed.). (1973). *Loneliness: The experience of emotional and social isolation*. Cambridge, MA: MIT Press.

WHO (1963). *International classification of diseases*. Tenth Revision (ICD 10).

Willis, S.L., & Belleville, S. (2016). Cognitive training in later adulthood. In K.W. Schaic & S.K. Willis (Eds.), *Handbook of the psychology of aging*, Eighth Edition (pp. 219–243). Cambridge, MA: Academic Press.

Wilkinson, P.J., & Coleman, P.G. (2010). Strong beliefs and coping in old age: A case-based comparison of atheism and religious faith. *Aging & Society*, 30, 337–361.

Windsor, T.D., Curtis, R.G., & Luszcz, M.A. (2015). Sense of purpose as a psychological resource for aging well. *Developmental Psychology*, 51, 975–986.

Wong, P. (1989). Personal meaning and successful aging. *Canadian Psychology*, 30, 516–525.

Wong, P., & Tomer, A. (2011). Beyond Terror and denial: The positive psychology of acceptance. *Death Studies*, 35, 99–106.

Wood, A.M., Froh, J.J., & Geraghty, W.A. (2010). Gratitude and well-being: A review and theoretical integration. *Clinical Psychology Review*, 30, 890–905.

Wood, W., & Runger, D. (2016). Psychology of habit. *Annual Review of Psychology*, 67, 289–314.

Wortman, C.B., & Silver, R.C. (1990). Successful mastery of bereavement and widowhood: A life course perspective. In P.B. Baltes & M.M. Baltes (Eds.), *Successful aging: Perspectives from the behavioral sciences* (pp. 225–264). New York, NY: Cambridge University Press.

Wrosch, C., & Heckhausen, J. (2002). Perceived control of life regrets: Good for young and bad for old adults. *Psychology and Aging*, 17, 340–350.

Wrosch, C., Bauer, I., & Scheier, M.F. (2005). Regret and quality of life across the adult span: The influence of disengagement and available future goals. *Psychology and Aging*, 20, 657–670.

Wrosch, C., Bauer, I., Miller, G.E., & Lupien, S. (2007). Regret intensity, diurnal cortisol secretion, and physical health in older individuals: Evidence for directional effects and protective factors. *Psychology and Aging*, 22, 319–330.

Yalom, I.D. (1980). *Existential psychotherapy*. New York, NY: Basic Books.

Yalom, I.D. (2008). *Staring at the Sun*. San Francisco, CA: Jossey-Bass.

Young, Y., Frick, K.D., & Phelan, E.A. (2009). Can successful aging and chronic illness coexist in the same individual? *Journal of the American Medical Directors Association*, 10, 87–92.

Index